FOOTPRINTS IN THE SAND OF CAREGIVING

Footprints in the Sand of Caregiving

Copyright © 2024 by Leandro (Lany) Maniwang Tapay

Published in the United States of America

ISBN	Paperback:	979-8-89091-440-8
ISBN	Hardback:	979-8-89091-441-5
ISBN	eBook:	979-8-89091-442-2

All rights reserved. No part of this publication may be reproduced, stored in a retrieval system or transmitted in any way by any means, electronic, mechanical, photocopy, recording or otherwise without the prior permission of the author except as provided by USA copyright law.

The opinions expressed by the author are not necessarily those of ReadersMagnet, LLC.

ReadersMagnet, LLC 10620 Treena Street, Suite 230 | San Diego, California, 92131 USA
1.619. 354. 2643 | www.readersmagnet.com

Book design copyright © 2024 by ReadersMagnet, LLC. All rights reserved.

Cover design by Andrew Patrick Crawford
Interior design by Daniel Lopez

FOOTPRINTS IN THE SAND OF CAREGIVING

A soul's reflections on its solitary walk on the seashore of a lonely island of caregiving

By
Leandro (Lany) Maniwang Tapay

Former Diocesan Director
The Pontifical Mission Societies in the United States
Diocese of Columbus, Ohio

ReadersMagnet, LLC

Lovingly dedicated to Delores Jean Tapay, my beloved wife, whose illness brought us to our knees.

My Dear Reader,

Before you read this book, I would like you to know about my wife, Delores Jean Tapay, to whom this book is lovingly dedicated.

In my opinion, she is the most beautiful woman in the world – both inside and outside. She is a very caring, loving and positive person. She spent many years caring for the sick. Everyone in the hospital where she worked loved and admired her character and spirituality.

Sadly and understandably, when she had to be confined to a bed because of illness, it altered her way of seeing things. She lost her filters; she tells you exactly what is in her heart.

At times, her frustration causes her to throw verbal rocks at people. Being constantly at her side, I am often hit by those imaginary rocks.

My dear reader, I want you to know that my experiences in caring for her, which I describe in this book, are by no means ugly characterizations of my wife, nor are they putdowns or complaints.

The caregiving experiences I share are my raw responses to the struggles I face daily (24/7) in taking care of my wife.

I could not survive in this caregiving journey without God's love and mercy. I cannot see the days ahead but I know that God is and will be with me.

May the reflections I share serve as tiny flickers of light to those who are stumbling while going through the dark valleys in the journey of life.

Thanks in advance for reading "Footprints in the Sands of Caregiving." May God bless you and your loved ones. Praise the Lord!

Sincerely yours in Mary of Mount Carmel,
Lany

TABLE OF CONTENTS

FOREWORD - Rev. Father Terry Tapay, SDB xiii
FOREWORD - Rev. Father Dennis Nacorda xv
ACKNOWLEDGEMENTS xvii
PROLOGUE xix
PREFACE xxi
INTRODUCTION - Mary Kate Crawford Mbengue xxiii
INTRODUCTION - Paula Coleman Black, DDS xxv

CHAPTER 1 1
CHAPTER 2 6
CHAPTER 3 11
CHAPTER 4 17
CHAPTER 5 22
CHAPTER 6 27
CHAPTER 7 32
CHAPTER 8 37
CHAPTER 9 43
CHAPTER 10 47
CHAPTER 11 53
CHAPTER 12 58
CHAPTER 13 64
CHAPTER 14 69
CHAPTER 15 74
CHAPTER 16 79
CHAPTER 17 84
CHAPTER 18 89
CHAPTER 19 94
CHAPTER 20 98
CHAPTER 21 103
CHAPTER 22 108
CHAPTER 23 113
CHAPTER 24 118

BIOGRAPHY 121

Most Rev. Dr. George Antonysamy
Archbishop of Madras and Mylapore

MS/ABS/24/02 Chennai, 09 January 2024

Addressing participants in the General Assembly of The Pontifical Academy for Life on the occasion of the 20th Anniversary of its founding, Pope Francis stated, "In our societies we find the tyrannical dominion of an economic logic that excludes and sometimes kills, of which so many today are victims, beginning with our elderly…Therefore, poor health and disability are never a good reason for excluding or, worse, for eliminating a person; and the most serious privation that an elderly person undergoes is not the weakening of the body and the disability that may ensue, but abandonment and exclusion, the privation of love."

The growing technological advancement and its modern approach towards human life present certain natural human limitations and even old age and the challenges it entails to be a disability and a criterion to be excluded from society. It appears as if the world could accept and guarantee life only for those who are powerful, healthy, and capable of contributing to society. There is clearly the loss of the sense of God, and there is also the tendency to lose the sense of man his dignity and his life, which Pope St. John Paul II calls, 'the culture of death' in his encyclical *Evangelium Vitae* while referring to the evils of abortion and euthanasia.

The conventional understanding of pain and suffering is that it is bad, evil and something to be avoided. While it may be arguably true, what shall we do with persons for whom suffering and agony are their sole companions? How to respond to aging spouses who grapple with loneliness, disability and illnesses? In the modern era, it is quite amazing to see married couples who being faithful to their marital promises jog along to the sunset of their life. From welcoming Christian vocation to the sacrament of matrimony to joyfully sharing the challenges of old age it offers them, the brave example of the elderly couples has to be applauded. Unfortunately, though, the world we live in does not appreciate them. We do not consider them worthy of respect and dignity. We have created a 'throw-away' culture which is now spreading. (*Evangelii Gaudium*, n. 53)

In this context, 'Footprints in the Sand of caregiving' is not only a testimony but an invitation to our change of perspective towards the infirm and those needing love and care. Before looking out let us look within! Let us look at our own families! And Lany for me is a beacon of hope! I have always observed Lany a practical person, perceiving God's hand through personal experiences that await one's docile response. By caring for his infirm wife, he has learned to see the other side of suffering and inability, which offers an invitation to love. We can understand reading this book, how he conceptualizes pain, loneliness, marital fidelity, call to service and many other Christian virtues, and literally makes an ideal journey with the author who stimulates the reader to pronounce an individual response to possible situations like these. I see in Lany a faithful Catholic, a caring spouse and a subtle catechist who, through personal experiences that taught him who Christ is and what Christian vocation could be, makes the best use to replicate it into teaching manuals for others. His 'faith pedagogy' must be appreciated.

While congratulating him for this personal testimony, I invite spouses to seek and find joy in matrimony in good and bad, in sickness and health, by renewing their promises for each other that grow and mature in old age.

With every good wish, I remain

In Christ our Lord,

+ George Antonysamy
Archbishop of Madras-Mylapore

Archbishop's House, # 41, San Thome High Road, Chennai 600 004.
+91 - 44 - 2464 1102 / 2464 0833 +91 - 44 - 2464 1999 Email: abpmmsec@gmail.com / archmsmlsec@gmail.com

FOREWORD

By

Rev. Father Terry Tapay, SDB
Thailand

I thank Manong Lany for giving me a space and special privilege to express my feelings about his book "Footprints in the Sand of a Caregiver". As I was reading the book I was reminded of what I tell people the meaning of "retired". I told them to be tired again in one way or another. In the book "Footprints in the Sand of a Caregiver" I observed the secret of the inner strength amidst the physical tiredness. I believe that Manong Lany's secret is what St. Paul wrote to the Galatians "For when we are in union with Christ Jesus neither circumcision or the lack of it makes any difference; what matters is faith that works through love". (Gal 5:6)

As his younger brother I believe that he was the instrument of God that I am now a Salesian Missionary priest. When I was small my mother often wrote letters to him when he was still a seminarian asking advice what to do with me who was becoming naughty. One day he came home and that very day he brought me to Don Bosco Boys Town, a center famous for reforming naughty children. I observed his dedication in giving us a solid foundation for a good and successful life. After my elementary graduation I asked his advice about my becoming a priest. He arranged everything for me. I thank him very much.

When I was reading the book in its totality I was pondering at the anecdotes, events and experiences in parallel with my 50 years this year of my missionary life. This book encouraged me of my missionary principle. "No choice of work, no choice of people and no choice of place." I am sure that they who will read this book will have a Eucharistic meaning of life. "This is my body which will be given up for you."

FOREWORD

By Rev. Father Dennis Nacorda

New Zealand

This book unfolds a testament to the profound journey of Uncle Lany in caring for Auntie Jean who has grown weak under the burden of years.

In the tapestry of life, love weaves a thread binding two souls together, forming a bond that transcends the ordinary and withstands the tests of time. This love is the unwavering strength and resilience required in life's unpredictable journey.

The role of a caregiver is profound. The challenges demand a deep reservoir of compassion and an unyielding commitment. Obviously a myriad of emotions accompany such a time — love, devotion, frustration and at times, even despair. This journey needs to be navigated with faith, grace, understanding and an unshakeable commitment to the well-being of a loved one.

Caring for someone dependent on us in almost everything, is a deeply compassionate duty. Literally meaning "to suffer with," compassion aims for the alleviation of the condition that afflicts another. St. Augustine states, "what is compassion but a fellow-feeling in our hearts for another's misery, which compels us to come to help by every means in our power?" (City of God, Book IX, Chapter 5) Jesus went beyond that by entering our humanity and showing us how to face such trials. His risen presence strengthens us to be faithful and compassionate.

Essentially, this book narrates a story of the transformative power of compassion. Compassion is a choice made daily in the small, seemingly mundane tasks that constitute the fabric of daily life. It is the quiet strength that propels Uncle Lany forward, even when faced with seemingly insurmountable obstacles. This book illuminates the beauty in the ordinary acts of caregiving, emphasizing the profound impact these have had on both Uncle Lany and Auntie Jean. The love and care one invests are transformative forces, shaping not only the other person's world but also the landscape of one's own heart.

This book is a beacon of hope, a source of wisdom, and a testament to the extraordinary power of compassion in the face of adversity. It offers solace, guidance, and encouragement to those embarking on the sacred journey of caring for a loved one — a journey, though challenging, is also rich with opportunities for growth and the deepening of love

ACKNOWLEDGMENTS

I would like to thank:
- Patrick Andrew Crawford, my grandson, Founder and CEO of Blackletter Studio, for the cover design.
- His Excellency, George Antonysamy, the Archbishop of Madras - Mylapore, India – a former Apostolic Nuncio to Guinea, Liberia, Gambia, Sierra Leon; the Reverend Terry Maniwang Tapay, SDB, my brother, a Salesian Missionary in Thailand; the Rev. Father Dennis Tapay Nacorda, my nephew, from the Archdiocese of Wellington, New Zealand – for their foreword.
- Mary Kate Crawford, my granddaughter and Dr. Paula Coleman Black, DDS, my former student, for their introduction.
- Tim Puet of the Catholic Times, Diocese of Columbus for his initial editing guidance.
- To Father, God, whose plan for my life never alters, Whose steadfast love and mercy are new every morning.

PROLOGUE

Caregiving is a challenging mission.

Caregiving is a like a lonely island.

Withdrawn from my previous routines, lifestyle and social activities to focus on caregiving, I feel isolated and disconnected.

In my loneliness and desperation, from the bottom of my heart, I cry to the Lord and the Lord answers me saying: *"My steadfast love never ceases; my mercies never come to an end; they are new every morning; great is my faithfulness"* (Lamentations 3: 22 -23).

What a wonderful promise of God! When I am tempted to wallow in the mud of self-pity, I turn my gaze to the Lord. When I become depressed and distressed, I cling to the hope of His unceasing love.

PREFACE

God uses everything – the good and the bad – to show His glory.

Your pain has a purpose. Your problems, struggles, heartaches, and hassles lead to one end – the glory of God,

When problems and pain come your way, remember that nothing comes to your life (the good and the not so good) without God's approval.

Rather than complain or cry about the challenges you face, consider them as opportunities to give glory to God.

Ask God to give you the patience and strength to bear your burdens in a way that will honor God.

Don't focus on the trials, instead focus your gaze on Jesus hanging on the cross.

"Many are the afflictions of the righteous, but the Lord *delivers him out of them all*" (Psalm 14:19). Scriptures says.

INTRODUCTION

By

Mary Kate Crawford Mbengue

After almost 50 years of working, Lany, my fun-loving, peaceful grandfather, was expecting leisure and enjoyment during his retirement. Becoming my grandmother's full time caregiver was not what he had envisioned and certainly not what he wanted to do alone. As Lany puts it, these were the cards he was dealt, and he had no choice but to play the cards that were in his hands.

Lany, devout Catholic and husband, gets really personal in *Footprints in the Sand of Caregiving*. He is able to pour out his heart and mind on the following pages. His reflections of taking care of his wife, my grandmother, are difficult to read at times. Lany respectfully writes about her becoming disabled and no longer being able to care for herself in any capacity. Bound to a wheelchair, he must do everything for her which he writes about in great detail…often humorously: "In an instant, I became a cook, a housekeeper, a laundry man, a nurse, a physical therapist and many other titles like denture coordinator or enema specialist. I became the proverbial "Jack of all trades – master of none".

Is she the appreciative patient who feels embarrassed when she receives more than she can give? Nay! No matter how difficult she is or the extreme pain she causes him, he refuses to treat her unkindly or give up on her acknowledging the pain and loss of dignity that *she* has gone through instead. Even through the challenges each chapter discusses, Lany's faith and love for Christ shines through. He always brings every experience back to Christ teaching his readers no struggle is meaningless.

Despite Lany's battling with the stresses of his new role of 24/7 caregiver to his wife, Lany knows this is not how things will end for him. Ever faithful servant, Lany accepts God's will for his life because even though he knows it's so hard sometimes, the heavenly rewards are greater. Like Job, Lany reminds his readers the importance of remaining calm and to continue to praise Jesus for all his blessings.

This is a raw account of a man who is dealing with an unexpected time in his life. He mourns his old life and struggles with the guilt and pain of being a caregiver to his beloved wife who takes out her frustration and pain on him on a daily basis. So many readers can relate to this. When Lany struggles, he always goes back to Jesus and his teachings. Through these accounts, Lany is teaching us a very valuable lesson about our own lives: "If I follow Jesus, I can't be angry with my care receiver." for Lany reminds us that Jesus never said if you follow him, you will have no troubles. No matter how deep our faith is, we are never guaranteed a trouble free life. Instead, Jesus said, "If you follow me, take up your cross daily."

INTRODUCTION

By

Paula Coleman Black, DDS

It is with the utmost honor and humility I introduce you to *Footprints in the Sand of Caregiving.*

Leandro Tapay was a colleague of my mother and was my guidance counselor during my time at London High School in the late 1970s and early 1980s. This was a time when the quality of an educational system began to be measured by objective ratings and the opportunities afforded by Title IX were turning heads. In many ways, these were unchartered waters. A response by some, understandably, was 'this isn't how we typically do this or that.' Lany had a gift for not buying into such framework thinking and chose not to see such boundaries. This carried over to how he advised and counseled his colleagues and students.

Many of the directions I have chosen in my life have been apart from what many would consider the norm yet they have seemed so natural to me. Some examples: I discerned that

I wanted to be a dentist when I was in junior high school. Remember, the times – it was 'ok' for a girl to go to college, but not so much for a girl to go to graduate school, let alone dental school. With Mr. Tapay's suggestion, I visited OSU's College of Dentistry the spring of my *freshman* year of high school. (Ponder this – in today's age, it's customary to make a college visit for an undergraduate program during one's senior year). At the beginning of my sophomore year of high school, the 'boys' golf team needed one more player. I wasn't the lowest scoring golfer, but I could golf. Yes, I played on the 'boys' team and varsity lettered three years! One of my classes my senior year was Accounting 1. This year long class was self-paced and the material came very easy to me. By the end of the first semester, I had completed the entire year. I ended up completing the coursework for Accounting 2 the second semester of the year with a month to spare.

Why are these three examples important to me? Obviously, being accepted to and graduating from dental school were major accomplishments and provided me with an amazing career. But with that career, I was able to help people. Dentistry is something about which people have many society-driven opinions, but I believe my patients benefited from my care and concern. Golf is a sport I have thoroughly loved. Being able to play in the format I did helped me learn how to understand and to get along with many types of people. This skill helped me swim in a male-dominated graduate program and career. What is so special about finishing the accounting coursework? Obviously, it wasn't the easy or typical way. Business classes like these are very important but I had limited windows of opportunity and time. Yet, learning such information definitely proved to be useful when I became a small business owner, who ran a dental practice, negotiated business loans, and managed an office building. A common comment I've encountered was 'dental school doesn't teach about running a business'. True, but it's not true to assume a dentist doesn't know anything about business.

Lany's guidance and way of thinking helped lay a solid foundation of confidence for me and for many others. He didn't see boundaries and he strived for developing one's potential. He truly believed in his students. Lany's writing lays a similar foundation for those who have found themselves caring for a loved one in times past or who are in the midst of doing so now.

Many things in life are not easy and caregiving is one of them. Lany's sharing of his genuine heart and his incredible witness of faith in God offers purpose and value to caregiving and to living life.

CHAPTER 1

ALL IS WELL WITH MY SOUL

After 49 years of working with the public (35 years as a guidance counselor at London, Ohio, High School and 14 years as director for the Pontifical Mission Societies in the United States in the Diocese of Columbus, Ohio), I was looking forward to a happy and enjoyable retirement.

The word *retirement* sounded peaceful and relaxing; no more deadlines to meet, no more staff meetings to attend; no more setting of the alarm clock; having more time for coffee in the morning on my porch, admiring the flowers and watching butterflies of various colors and varieties in my yard.

But that was not meant to be. Instead, God gave me a third job: a mission of 24/7 caregiving for my beloved wife, Delores Jean Tapay, beginning on June 19, 2020.

Coincidentally, just as I was about to retire from working for the diocese, my wife became disabled. Her knees gave out.

I had applied for my first two jobs, sending prospective employers a resume to prove that I had the qualifications, education and training needed to be successful in those jobs.

The third job did not require an application or a resume. I did not have the qualifications, education or training for it. And in this job, I cannot have a vacation, I cannot quit and I cannot retire.

But there is nothing I can do about it. Those are the cards dealt to me and I have no choice but to play the cards that are in my hands.

Relaxing, peaceful retirement was my plan, but it was not God's. God is not done with me yet.

She can stand up but can no longer walk, even with the help of a walker or a cane. She is completely dependent on me. She cannot go to the bathroom by herself. I have to help her stand and guide her to her wheelchair. In the bathroom, I have to help her stand and guide her to the commode.

When we were purchasing a wheelchair for her, Dr. Stock her principal physician, said she was going to lose her leg muscles and would not be able to walk again, and she was right. After a few months of using the wheelchair her leg muscles became weaker.

For several years, she took pain medication by mouth whenever it was needed (which was often), and every two months she received treatment to ease her pain.

She received an injection in her kneecap and the medication slowly destroyed her knee ligaments. At a certain point, knee replacement no longer was an option.

I remembered my brother-in-law, Jerry Crumpler, saying that when life goes sour, "If you get lemons, make lemonade."

"I will be drinking a lot of lemonade in the coming years," I told myself.

I always enjoy talking with Jerry. He is a well-rounded man who can talk about almost any subject and tells many jokes.

Jerry is a self-made man. He started as a truck driver, delivering gasoline for Gulf Oil. Between deliveries, he volunteered to help with paperwork in the office. His superiors took notice of this and of his ability to get along with people.

He was promoted to an office job, and whenever his assigned task was completed ahead of time, he volunteered to help others who were behind on their work.

"Jerry, why do you work so hard?" a co-worker asked him. "You are not being paid more by doing extra work."

His hard work paid off. He kept being promoted and retired as superintendent of the entire southern district of the United States for Chevron Oil, which had acquired Gulf and in turn was acquired at the time of his retirement by BP (British Petroleum). Gulf was founded and based in Pittsburgh and its brand still exists in the eastern United States.

Jerry's length of service and position with the company provided him with a notable retirement income.

"The gentleman who asked me why I was working extra time without pay remained stuck in the same job classification level and never got a promotion during his tenure with the company," Jerry said.

When I was writing this chapter, the Sunday Gospel reading was about Jesus' parable of the sower. This man scattered seeds and some fell on hard soil and did not germinate. Others fell on soil full of thistles and germinated, but were choked by the thistles. Others fell on rich soil, germinated and provided a good harvest. The seeds represent God's word and the soil is people's hearts.

The seed also could represent my two jobs at London and with the Diocese of Columbus. In both cases, the seed fell on rich soil because God put the right people and the right situations and events in place to accomplish His plan for my life.

"Life can be understood only in looking backward, but it must be lived forward," the philosopher Soren Kierkegaard said.

In looking back at my life, I can see the finger of God working to accomplish His plan for my life. I am always stunned at his orchestration.

I cannot see how my third job (24/7 caregiving) will turn out in the years ahead, but I know it is God's plan and because of it, I can move forward with confidence that all will be well.

Horatio Spafford was a successful Chicago lawyer; his 4-year-old son perished in the 1871 Chicago fire, which also devoured his substantial real estate investments. His business interests were hit heavily in the 1873 economic downturn.

He planned to travel to England with his family, but he sent his wife and four daughters ahead of him because of a zoning problem related to the fire and planned to join them later.

The ship carrying his wife and daughters collided with another ship and sank, killing all four daughters. His wife survived and sent him a telegram saying simply, "Saved alone." Shortly afterward, he traveled to England to be with his grieving wife.

On his way to England, in the area where his four daughters perished, he wrote a beautiful hymn titled
It Is Well with My Soul. Here is the first stanza:

> When peace like a river attendeth my way
> When sorrows like sea billows roll
> Whatever my lot, Thou has taught me to say
> It is well, it is well with my soul.

Whenever I pass through the troubled waters of life, the lyrics and melody of this song calm my soul, as they did for Mr. Spafford.

I commend my caregiving journey to our loving Father, accepting his plan for my life. To Him be the glory. I continue my journey as a 24/7 caregiver with this song in my heart.

CHAPTER 2

The pain of losing one's dignity

When I retired, I left my heart in the missions office at the Diocese of Columbus. I miss my coworkers at the Catholic Center; I miss my co- diocesan directors of the Pontifical Mission Societies in the United States; I miss the folks at the National Office in New York; I miss the missionaries around world who came to visit Columbus during mission appeals.

I praise and thank God for the opportunity of having served the Church in a unique way as a director of the Pontifical Mission Societies in the United States for the Diocese of Columbus. I had been an honor and a privilege.

"You will not regret your decision to retire and take care of your wife." Deacon Tom Berg, Jr., the diocesan chancellor, told me when I told him about my situation home. My wife became physically disabled. Her knees gave up on her.

In an instant, I became a cook, a housekeeper, a laundry man, a nurse, a physical therapist and many other titles like denture coordinator or enema specialist. I became a proverbial "Jack of all trades – master of none".

Though I do not have an aptitude for cooking (I do not like to cook), in a few months I mastered the art of cooking sloppy joe, chili, taco, sour kraut.

"Your mashed potatoes is out of this world." My wife told me. I did not think it was sarcasm.

Not long after I became a caregiver, I became more aware that there are more tips and advises for caregivers than care receivers. It seems that people are more concerned with caregivers than care receivers.

For several years when the Ohio State University Newman Center was still managed and run by the Paulist Fathers, I was blessed with the opportunity to serve in the teams that coordinated the Masses there and the team that brought Holy Communion to the Catholic patients at the Ohio State Hospital. I considered it an honor and a privilege to serve on those teams.

I thank God for the blessings. I always thought that I was more blessed than the patients with whom I visited.

Some of the patients were disabled seniors from nursing homes. I enjoyed visiting with them. "I truly enjoyed talking with you and your visit made my day." An elderly lady from Delaware, Ohio told me, one evening.

"It was Jesus that made your day." I thought to myself, but I did not tell her what I thought. Instead, I said: "Me, too".

When I looked at the disabled seniors and when I listened to their stories, I felt their pain – both physical and psychological; they felt that they are worthless; they felt they lost their dignity.

Most care-receiver feel they have lost their dignity. In our culture that emphasizes productivity, the weak and the vulnerable become rejects; they are obstacles in the pursuit of money and convenience.

In previous civilizations, people worshiped idols; they sacrificed their babies to their gods. Our current culture, also worship idols; the god of money and the god of convenience.

Our current culture sacrifices our babies to the god of convenience, and warehouses our old people in nursing homes.

The number of babies aborted in America had surpassed the number of Jews murdered by Adolf Hitler during WWII. And we take pride in saying that we live in a Christian nation.

Nowadays there some conversations going around about the idea of mercy killing. Do you remember the notable Dr. Jack Kevorkian? His idea is floating even in the medical community.

"Lany, you are getting old! Don't climb up the roof anymore; because if you fall, the doctors will not do much to save you; because of your age the doctors will tranquilize you and let you go peacefully." My doctor told me during one of annual physical checkup.

Was my doctor joking? I do not know. I did not ask him. What do you think?

At the office after my Urologist examined my rectum: "Lany, you have an enlarged prostate gland. But you do not have cancer; I can assure you that you will die from a prostate cancer; but I tell you, had you have cancer in your prostate, because of your age (80 at that time), I would not do anything heroic about it; I would just keep you comfortable." My Urologist explained to me.

"You are fired!" I thought to myself. I thought of pointing my index finger to his face. Though I was very angry at him, I did not do it. I did not want to lose my dignity. I tried to stay calm, but I left the office furious at his attitude toward old people.

After that incident, I changed my urologist.

Not long ago, I asked a neighbor how her mother was doing in the nursing home.

"She is OK, but if her condition remains the way it is, I'm afraid none of her money will be left for us children when she dies," she said with a laugh. I did not think it was funny.

I thought of the parable of the prodigal son. The young man asked his father for his inheritance. What the son did was a first-class insult to the father. According to the custom of that time, inheritances were given to sons only after the death of the father.

In effect, what the son was saying to his father was, "Dad, I wish you were dead!"

When my mother in the Philippines had a stroke, my brother wrote me and said, "I am remodeling the house to accommodate our mother's needs (There was no texting at the time). In my town of Balilihan in Bohol province in the Philippines, there are no nursing homes. The family takes care of the disabled and elderly at home.

Back to care receivers: perhaps the greatest psychological pain my wife suffers because of her disability, is the feeling that she is losing her dignity.

Before she became disabled, she was dignified and beautiful and took good care of her looks.

Now she is frustrated because she no longer can take care of herself the way she used to.

The thought of losing one's dignity is painful. To alleviate my wife's pain about this, I am trying my best to restore it in the ways I can.

I did not sell her car. It is still in the driveway although she no longer can drive. She still has her car keys and driver's license.

She still has her bank account, credit cards and checkbook. I told her that she could keep 100 percent of her Social Security and pension checks.

She is proud that she has a notable amount in her savings account. She is very protective of her bank account.

CHAPTER 3

The gut-wrenching cry of loneliness

Caregiving on a 24/7 basis is a challenging mission; and I can neither quit nor retire. I am afraid that if I do, I might end up as Jonah did. And I do not want to be thrown into a dark and stormy sea and be swallowed by a big fish.

Do you remember what happened to Jonah when he disobeyed God?

God told Jonah to preach repentance to the people of Nineveh concerning their sinfulness and to tell them to change their ways, otherwise, God's wrath would fall on them.

"If I preach to them and they would repent and nothing would happen to them, they will call me a false prophet. I am not going to preach there," Jonah said to himself.

So instead of boarding a boat for Nineveh, he boarded one going in the opposite direction. That boat encountered a severe storm in the middle of the sea and its crew suspected that the storm was triggered by a sinner who was a passenger among them. This was a common belief at that time.

While the crew was determining who the culprit was, Jonah confessed that he was a prophet and asked the crew to throw him into the dark, stormy sea to save the boat from sinking.

As a caregiver, I am like Jonah. It is as if I have been thrown into the dark, stormy sea of life waiting to be swallowed by a big fish. Like Jonah, I am floating on the seas of life.

I miss interacting with people because I cannot go out as I used to. I notice that I have developed the tendency to talk to people more than before as a way of overcompensating for my isolation. I engage in conversation with almost anyone I encounter. I need to be careful not to make a fool of myself and lose my dignity.

Thanks to God, I found something to mitigate my loneliness. Through Facebook, I have gotten in touch with some of my former students and faculty members at London (Ohio) High School, where I worked for 35 years.

I am amazed at their warm response to my posts. Through connecting with former students and colleagues, I feel connected to the outside world.

It is very gratifying to hear my former students' stories about their journeys in life. Most of them have been very successful, becoming doctors, nurses, lawyers, priests and so on. Many already are grandparents and have retired.

"Mr. T, I am now a lawyer. In high school, you told me that there is no money in playing the piano," wrote Mary Ann, an excellent piano player and member of the high school band. She plays the organ for her church.

"My words mattered!" I thought. "Wow! I hope I did not ruin any lives by what I said to former students."

Jake, another former student, wrote, "Mr. T, I just got out from prison. You told me that if I did not change my behavior, I would end up in prison."

I did not ask Jake the circumstances of his incarceration. Instead, I wrote back, "I praise the Lord for your new freedom; always remember that God does not love you more when you are being good, nor does God love you less when you are not so good. His love for you has no condition. God loves you, period. Thanks for sharing your situation with me. It means a lot to me."

I have moved from place to place several times, but I never felt lonely until becoming a caregiver.

Somehow, the pain of loneliness that I endured more than seven decades ago when I left home for the first time, is creeping again into my life. It is like a small animal gnawing at the edges of my joy and peace.

I am not alone in this feeling. Recent research shows that the cry of loneliness is prevalent in our society.

If we stop and listen, we could hear that cry on loneliness from an abandoned child in an orphanage, or from a lonely and elderly mother in a nursing home whose children are too busy to visit, write or call.

If we stop and listen, we could hear the cry of loneliness in prison cells from prisoners who long for to be freed.

If we visit a hospital, we could hear the cry of loneliness from hospitalized persons dying of cancer and other diseases.

If we pay attention to our conversations with other people, we could hear the cry of loneliness from women whose husbands left them for younger women.

If we walk in neighborhoods with manicured lawns in suburban America, we could hear the cry of loneliness, from aging homecoming queens with shattered dreams.

The cry of loneliness comes in various colors, shapes and forms. It does not respect age, gender or social status; it comes from the poor and the rich; from married people and single people; from those who have failed and those who have succeeded.

But the most gut-wrenching cry of loneliness did not come from an orphanage. It did not come from a nursing home, a hospital or a prison cell. It came from a hill – the hill of Calvary.

The most gut-wrenching cry of loneliness did come from an orphan, or from a person dying of cancer, or from a woman left by her husband, or from an orphan, or from a caregiver, or from a prisoner.

The gut-wrenching cry of loneliness came from Jesus, when He was dying on the cross.

Like the scapegoat of old which was left in the wilderness to die with the sins of the community dumped into it, Jesus the sin-bearer, was left alone at Calvary.

Jesus felt abandoned and said so, because the sins of all humanity from the beginning to the end of the world were dumped on Him.

Every lie ever told, every object ever coveted, every promise ever broken was placed on Jesus' shoulders. On Calvary, Jesus became sin (2 Corinthians 5:21).

Jesus felt so alone because only He could do what He was going to do. Only Jesus could redeem the world.

Sin and God do not mix. The Most Holy God cannot look at sin, so when the sins of the world were placed on Jesus, the Father turned His gaze away from the Son. Jesus felt abandoned by the Father.

It was more than Jesus could take. He withstood the beating, the nailing to the cross, the mockery and the Apostles abandoning Him. Jesus did not retaliate when thugs hurled insults at Him. He did not resist when nails pierced His hands and feet.

But when God turned His face away from Jesus, it was more than Jesus could handle; the Father turning His gaze away from Jesus broke the camel's back. His heart was broken to pieces and He cried "My God, my God, why have you forsaken me?]" (Matthew 27:46).

"My God!" The wail came from Jesus' parched lips. Jesus' holy heart was broken. Jesus, the sin-bearer, screamed as He wandered in the eternal wasteland.

From Jesus came words screamed by all of us who walk in the desert of loneliness. The pain caused by the feeling of being abandoned by God can make anyone cry from his or her gut.

Be thankful if your heart has never been broken by loneliness, or if you have not felt that your life was dark and that God seemed far away. Count your blessings; pray that you may be spared the terrible pain of loneliness.

If you are now struggling with loneliness, know that God has felt infinitely more than you are feeling.

Picture Jesus, with His eyes misting and with His bruised hands wiping your tears away.

Even if Jesus seems to offer no answer to your pain, even if He may not solve your problem, Jesus, who was once alone understands your situation.

CHAPTER 4

I do not want to be with the goats

Job. I like the guy's attitude. Job was a wealthy man with a large family who lived in the land of Uz.

"Hi Satan, look at Job. The guy is so good there is none like him on earth," God told Satan.

Satan responded, "Yeah, because you bless him, you made him prosper. If I take away his possessions, for sure he will curse you."

"You are wrong, Satan. Job will never curse me. Go ahead, take away his possessions and you will see that he is not going to curse me," God challenged Satan.

While Job was relaxing one day, a messenger came to tell him, "Job, bad news! The Sabeans stole all your herd of oxen and donkeys; the Sabeans also killed the herd attendants."

Before Job could digest the bad news, another messenger arrived and said, "Job, the Chaldeans stole all your sheep and they killed the shepherds."

Before the second messenger could finish talking, a third messenger told Job his house had burned down, killing Job's sons and daughters who were partying there.

The news could blow up any man's brain, but instead, Job remained calm and worshiped God, saying, *"**God gives and God takes away. Blessed be God!**"*

Job is my model. Before I became a caregiver, God blessed me with a wonderful job as director of the Pontifical Mission Societies in the United States for the Diocese of Columbus, Ohio.

The blessings of the position were far beyond anyone could expect or imagine – attending daily Mass (serving often) at St. Joseph Cathedral; praying the Chaplet of Divine Mercy with other diocesan employees at 3 p.m.; hosting missionaries who were invited to participate in the MCP (Missionary Cooperation Plan) program.

On top of these blessings, my wonderful friend Father Ramon Owera, who at the time was administrator of Columbus St. Elizabeth Church, visited me every month and heard my confession in my office.

After confession, we went to lunch at Due Amici Ristorante near my office. His company – along with baked salmon, an Italian dessert, a sip of white Italian wine and cappuccino – was the highlight of my month.

God spoiled me with His blessings before I became a caregiver. Like Job, I praise the Lord in good times and in the not so good times.

Caregiving 24/7 is a very heavy cross to carry. God has given me many crosses before, but caregiving is the heaviest of all. It is making me a grouchy old man. I am becoming more impatient, like a time bomb about to explode.

Caregiving also makes the dark side of me come out. Every time I am scolded (which is often) for my inability to deliver to expectations, my blood boils. I get very angry.

"When you get angry, I am scared of you," my care receiver often reminds me.

When angry, I tend to shout, slam doors and pout. I hate this dark side of me and am trying to correct it, but sadly, am making only a tiny dent in it. Since I became a caregiver, I confess the same sins over and over. I have a long way to go before I become a smiling caregiver.

Since my care receiver completely relies on me, I am often in demand. Some of my care receiver's demands for help need immediate response, like going to the bathroom. In this matter, I render help right away; I do not like to clean up the mess.

It is ugly. I know I do the things I do not want to do and do not do the things I should do, such as being kind and understanding. Have you ever been ugly?

If you have been ugly, then you know what I mean. If you have not, count your blessings and pray that God spares you from it.

I know I should do my caregiving task with a smile. But it is difficult to smile while cleaning vomit and diarrhea. I saw nurses in hospitals doing dirty tasks with ease and comfort, but I have a weak stomach. I gag easily.

I cannot smile when my care receiver wakes me up at 2 a.m. and wants to me to help her shave her legs or to change the television channel.

Generally, I comply to my care receiver's demands without comments because I know from experience that derogatory comments could trigger "a third world war."

Some people say I do not practice tough love and should set boundaries, but I have a problem with strict boundaries. In doing so, I put myself up and my care receiver down, as though I am the master and she should do what I say.

I cannot do that. In my book, that is a cruel thing to do. Being disabled, her ego already is so depleted that treating her like a child is like putting salt to her wound. I want to do everything in my power to preserve her dignity.

So what I am to do? Cry to the Lord for help.

When I get scared, or when I feel the heavy weight of caregiving, I visit the garden of Gethsemane and spend a few minutes with Jesus, listening to Him begging the Father to take the cross away from Him, then accepting not what he wants, but what the Father wants.

This recalls a story I either heard or read about an American soldier who took care of a sick Japanese soldier in a POW camp in the Pacific during World War II.

The American made it a point to talk to the Japanese man every day.

"Yuri, do not worry about dying. When you die, you will meet Jesus," the American said to the man when he was dying.

"John, if Jesus is like you, I really would like to meet Him," the man responded.

I pray that our Father God will give me grace to perform my caregiving activities in such a manner that my care receiver can see Jesus in me. I know that this is a very high goal, like the proverbial "threading a camel into a needle's eye." But with God, everything is possible.

On judgement day, when Jesus will return to judge the living and the dead, He will separate those who are saved from those who are not; the sheep (the good) will be on His right and the goats (the bad) on the left. I do not want to be among the goats. Do you?

CHAPTER 5

I can't be angry at my care receiver

The other day, my care receiver woke me up at 3 a.m. demanding breakfast.

I thought that maybe she forgot that in a hospital, a nursing home or a hotel, breakfast is not served at 3 a.m. or maybe she thought that she was on a flight from America to Manila, where dinner is served at Manila time.

I went to the kitchen to get her a bowl of Cheerios, her favorite brand of breakfast cereal. My care receiver is a brand fanatic, especially when it comes to food.

When I offered her Cheerios, she said, "No, I want a hot breakfast. I want bacon, eggs and grits like those we used to order in Granny's restaurant at Sea Colony in Carolina Beach.

Granny's is famous for its home-cooked meals. "Make sure that the bacon is well-done and crispy," my care receiver emphatically said.

At 3 a.m., I believe that a few care givers would say: "Go to you know where!" Though I was very angry, I bit my tongue and opted for peace in the house.

If you were me, would you comply with such a demand?

"Why in heck could she wait till 6 a.m. to eat breakfast?" I asked myself. I was livid.

I am afraid that anger is becoming my dominant emotion. I was known by many as a calm guy, but since I became a caregiver, I get angry very easy. I am like a time bomb.

"Was Jesus ever angry?" I asked myself. I found the answer to my question in Scripture.

I found that Jesus was not a passive man holding a lamb and never raising his voice. Jesus was angry on many occasions.

I found that anger is not always a sin, but what we do with our anger determines whether it is a sin.

Many things should make us angry. We should be angry with injustice, violence, greed, poverty and death because they are not right. Anger at these is called "righteous anger." This is the anger God feels when he sees the evil that is so pervasive in our world.

Righteous anger over evil is good, but in our anger, we should not sin. We should not fight evil with evil. Jesus has shown us a better way. According to Jesus' example, when my caregiver throws a stone at me, I should not throw it back at her. Instead, I should show her compassion, understanding and love.

Yes, this is unfair. And yes, it could cost me. But only love can stop evil. And that is exactly what Jesus did.

When Jesus was angry with evil in the world, he never stooped to its level. In his anger, he did not sin.

We live in a broken world. The evidence of it is everywhere - kids starving, people dying, broken families, mental health problems, war, sickness, pain, death, to name a few. We are not OK. The world is not OK.

And Jesus was angry about it. We could see anger in Jesus' response to evil.

Jesus wept when his friend Lazarus died. He was so deeply moved by the death of his friend that he yelled, "Lazarus! Come out!" Jesus was mad at the human condition.

The Jewish leaders in Jesus' time valued adherence to the law more than caring for the people.

The law was established to help people stay in the right relationship with God and with one another. But the Jewish leaders missed the heart of the law in pursuit of strict adherence to it.

Jesus continually broke the extra rules that Jewish leaders put in to protect the law. That made them angry at Jesus.

Jesus healed sick people on the Sabbath in front of the Jewish leaders to show them that caring for people is more important than obeying the law. Jesus was angry with those who hindered people from getting closer to God.

Jesus loves children and promised punishment for those who harmed them. "Unless you become like a child, you cannot enter heaven," He proclaimed.

In one instance, the Apostles tried to take Jesus away from children. They thought there were bigger fish to fry. It was a big mistake. Jesus rebuked them.

God's heart is like this. God is deeply moved when a child is sick or hurt, lonely, in distress, abandoned, hungry or abused. Jesus was angry with those who neglected children.

He was angry with the Pharisees. They pretended to be good, but they messed up people's lives. They pretended that their lives were in order while ignoring the sinfulness of their heart.

Jesus did not come for the good guys; He came for sinners and the sick. Jesus was angry with those who were self-righteous.

Jesus was angry with those who had ulterior motives and self-ambition. He was angry with the Pharisees because they prayed loudly in public so people could praise them.

Jesus preferred the widow's pennies over the large bags of coins from the Pharisees.

I used to think that God was like a police officer who wants me to obey the laws, and when I don't, He gets me.

Now I believe that God is not really in favor of submissive people who just blindly follow him. I believe that God is more interested in my relationship with Him and with His relationship with His people.

God wants our hearts. Laws were established to bring us closer to Him. Jesus showed us this reality.

Jesus saw the facades that many people put up. He saw people doing right things for wrong reasons.

Jesus is more interested in what is going on in our hearts than what we portray outwardly. He is angry with people doing good things for selfish reasons.

Our own anger is directed to those who wrong us. We have every reason to be angry with those people. "They deserve it," we rationalize.

But that is not Jesus' way. We follow the God who gives us what we need instead of what we deserve. We deserve nothing.

Jesus modeled this for us. Jesus did not lash out, even though he had every right to do so.

We can be angry, but with righteous anger. We need to always remember that only on the cross was God's anger with us satisfied.

If I follow Jesus, I can't be angry with my care receiver.

CHAPTER 6

Jesus' wondrous gift – the gift of peace

"Oh no!" I said to myself when I felt my cell phone in my pocket vibrating. My suspicion was right. The call was from my care receiver, who was panicking because she had an urgent need to go to the bathroom.

"Come home right now!" she urged in a voice so loud I had to hold the phone a foot away from my right ear. I was tempted to tell her to call 911. But I thought that an urgent need to go the bathroom would not qualify as a 911 emergency.

So, I pulled out from the checkout lane at the Kroger store and left my basketful of groceries against the wall near the checkout section without telling an attendant.

I ran to my car and drove home with my hazard lights blinking. I was rehearsing what and how to tell the police officer if I got caught speeding. My car's speed needle was on 55 mph in a 45-mph zone.

In spite of my efforts, I arrived late. The damage was already done. I almost cursed, but I got hold of myself. "I wish

I were like Mother Teresa, who provided great care in doing this type of job," I thought. I have a weak stomach. I gag easily.

When things at home became stable, I drove back to the store to resume checking out my groceries. This time, I obeyed the speed limit.

By then, an attendant had returned the items in my basket to the shelves. I had to start over. I almost became a basket case.

My luck did not improve as the day progressed. There was another surprise waiting for me when I returned home. After I put the groceries away, I went to the basement to do the laundry and found the floor filled with water. The water tank heater was leaking.

When I saw the flooded floor, dollar signs were floating in my head. I had just replaced the four tires of my Mazda and now my home needed a water tank.

When I shared the situation with my care receiver, she said, "Why are you telling me this, you mean guy? You just want to worry me." I felt like I was being slapped in the face.

"Sorry, I am telling you about it because I do not like to leave you in the dark. I would like you to feel that you are still a part of the living in this valley of tears," I explained it to my care receiver, but it didn't help.

As the flow of my day slowed down a bit, while sipping my coffee, the invitatory antiphon of the Liturgy of the Hours / Office of Readings flashed through my mind: "*Come into the Lord's presence singing for joy.*"

Yes, to have joy I need to come into the Lord's presence. "Lord, I am about to explode. Help me!" I cried out.

A thought came to mind: "If God could close the lion's mouth for Daniel, could part the Red Sea for Moses, could make the sun still for Joshua, could put a baby in the old arms of Sarah, could raise Lazarus from the dead, then God can certainly take care of me."

Jesus never said, "If you follow me, you will have no troubles."

No matter how deep our faith is, we are never guaranteed a trouble-free life. Instead, Jesus said, "If you follow me, take up your cross daily."

Peace is what Jesus promised to give us. At the resurrection, the first word He uttered was "Peace".

The disciples were happy to see Jesus alive, but they were also apprehensive. They wondered what Jesus would do to them after what they did to Him.

Instead of protecting Jesus, they all ran and hid, except for John. The others abandoned Jesus at that time He needed them most. So they were waiting for Him to rebuke them or to scold them for what they had done to him three days earlier.

But the anvil did not drop. Instead, Jesus said to them, "Peace.". For the disciples, it was a welcome relief.

The peace that Jesus promised is not the absence of trouble. It does not mean no more sickness, no more war, no more suicide bombing, no more hunger.

It does not mean all around is calm, our health is good, our income is steady or our kids are well.

For most of us, life is rarely calm. In this broken world, trouble is the norm.

"I told you all this so that trusting me, you will be unshakable, assured and deeply in peace," Jesus said.

In this broken world, we will continue to experience difficulties. But "Take heart! I have conquered the world," Jesus said (John 16:33).

Jesus' peace is not only possible; it is what we can and should expect as Christians.

There was peace in the bunker at Auschwitz in World War II where St. Maximilian Kolbe died.

Father Kolbe was a Franciscan priest who willingly surrendered his life so another prisoner who was a husband and a father would survive.

Father Kolbe was among a group of prisoners sent to a starvation bunker in retaliation for another prisoner's escape attempt. After more than two weeks without food and water, he was not dead – instead, he was leading the others still alive in the bunker in joyfully singing hymns which were heard by the Nazi guards and the other prisoners in the camp.

In the middle of Auschwitz, which was hell on earth – in the midst of conflict and trouble unlike anything most of us ever will see or could imagine – the men in Father Kolbe's bunker were singing hymns. There was peace in that bunker. Such is the peace that only Jesus can give.

For some of us, conflict or trouble is happening on a large scale because of health matters, financial concerns or the death of a loved one. For some of us, it is on a smaller scale.

In whatever is happening in our lives, Jesus' words are spoken to us personally. "Peace be with you. Do not let your heart be troubled. Do not be afraid," Jesus tells us.

Jesus' peace comes to us precisely in the midst of trouble. It did for St. Paul; it did for St. Maximilian Kolbe. It did for a dear friend who died of cancer not long ago.

The same Lord who lived in them lives in you and in me. Jesus' words are not just words. Jesus wants to give us the gift of peace.

Lord, grant that our hearts be always open to receive your wondrous and transforming gift – the gift of peace.

CHAPTER 7

I say David's prayer when I feel abandoned by God

Last night, when I was writing this chapter, I watched a CNN documentary titled "What Happened to the American Mayor?" about the rise and fall of Rudy Giuliani, the former mayor of New York City.

He was a rich, famous and beloved lawyer who owned several apartment complexes and other real estate properties in the city.

Before he became mayor, he successfully prosecuted Mafia family leaders and other notorious criminals.

The events of Sept. 11, 2001 happened during his mayorship and he became popular by the manner in which he handled the tragedy. He made an unsuccessful bid for the U.S. presidency during the 2008 Republican primaries.

What happened to Rudy? His downward spiral started when he began working as former President Donald Trump's personal lawyer.

Giuliani was among 18 people (including Trump) who were indicted by the Fulton County, Georgia, district attorney on charges of conspiring to overturn the results of the 2020 presidential election.

Giuliani went to Trump's Mar-A-Lago mansion in Florida to ask him for help in paying Giuliani's legal bills; Trump refused.

Some people believe that Giuliani is going to sell his assets to pay for his legal defense. Even if he does, he still may not have enough and may have to declare bankruptcy and seek legal help from public defenders.

If this happens, it would be a sad "riches to rags" story. I cannot imagine how someone would cope with such a fall.

When I became a caregiver, in a small way and in a different way, I was put into something that in a small way resembles Rudy's situation.

It was as if my life was turned upside down. I miss dressing up in a coat and tie and going to the office every working day. I miss the interaction with missionaries and bishops from mission nations who come to Columbus during the mission appeal season.

I had a difficult time coping with the transition from working in public, which I enjoyed so much to working on a one-to-one was basis with my care receiver. The difference was so drastic that it shocked my system. It is as if my life screamed "System overload!"

As a caregiver I feel that everything I do is unfinished business. I am called to duty more often than I can handle it. I am often overwhelmed by the needs of my care receiver.

When my name is called, I have to stop whatever I am doing. Quite often, my bathroom routine is interrupted in the middle; most of the time, the process is aborted altogether.

I think of firefighters. When the alarm sounds, they stop whatever they are doing, rush toward the firefighter's pole and slide down to the fire truck.

Sometimes I feel that the burden of caregiving is too heavy to carry. In those moments of discouragement, I cry out to the Lord to help me.

When I do, it is as if tiny flickering lights appear in the darkness of my life. They appear to me in the form of incidents in Jesus' life found in Scriptures.

The other day, the light that flickered was ***"I am giving you a new commandment; love one another as I have loved you"*** (John 13:34).

How can we love as Jesus loved? Jesus was perfect and we are not. Jesus knows it. But although we cannot love as He loved, we are all called to try.

Jesus showed us the importance of loving others in the story of Zacchaeus.

Zacchaeus was small-statured (like me) and a tax collector. In Jesus' time, tax collectors were considered thieves and sinners.

One day, Zach heard that Jesus was coming to town. He wanted to see Jesus. But because he was a small guy, he was afraid that because of the big crowd, he would miss the sight of Jesus passing by.

So to be sure he would not miss seeing Jesus, he climbed on a sycamore three near the road in which Jesus was traveling.

When Jesus passed by the sycamore tree, He looked up and saw Zacchaeus.

"Zacchaeus, come down. I would like to have lunch with you in your house," Jesus said.

"Oh no! My wife is going to kill for inviting a stranger for lunch without telling her," Zacchaeus probably thought.

Jesus was being kind to the small man in the tree. Other people might have ignored Zacchaeus. But Jesus did not.

Not only did Jesus notice Zacchaeus, He spent the whole day with him.

As a result, several "good people" were upset with what Jesus was doing.

"Why would Jesus spend time with a sinner when there are many good people around town?" they asked themselves.

"Hey Jesus, that guy is a con man! You are wasting your time with a crook," they may have thought. But they did not have the courage to tell their thoughts to Jesus.

It was a good thing that they did not do so; otherwise, Jesus probably would have rebuked them sternly.

Jesus dealt with Zacchaeus the way He did because Jesus knew how loving kindness could transform

Zacchaeus' heart.

Likewise, we have the opportunity to share God's love with others through kindness.

An old saying goes "A tiny drop of honey can catch more flies than a gallon of vinegar."

I wonder how I ever could carry on my mission as a caregiver without faith.

There are times when I feel I am abandoned by God, or that God does not care or does not hear my prayers.

When I do, I say David's prayer:

Psalm 13

¹How long wilt thou forget me, O LORD? forever? how long wilt thou hide thy face from me?

² How long shall I take counsel in my soul, having sorrow in my heart daily? how long shall mine enemy be exalted over me?

³ Consider and hear me, O LORD my God: lighten mine eyes, lest I sleep the sleep of death;

⁴ Lest mine enemy say, I have prevailed against him; and those that trouble me rejoice when I am moved.

⁵ But I have trusted in thy mercy; my heart shall rejoice in thy salvation.

⁶ I will sing unto the LORD, because he hath dealt bountifully with me.

CHAPTER 8

Jesus expects honesty, not perfection from us

"Why not develop the muscles in your arms like Mark?" my care receiver asked me one day as I struggled to transfer her from her wheelchair to her bed.

Mark is my care receiver's well-built, muscular hair stylist, a much bigger, much taller and much younger man than I am. He probably is in his late 30s or early 40s. He is a very kind man. He helps my care receiver get into our car every time we go to his salon to have her hair fixed. My care receiver wishes that I was big, strong and muscular.

"For heaven's sake, I am an 86-year-old man!" I thought when she asked about my arm muscles. I did not say anything to her because I did not want to start an argument. Past experiences have taught me when to fight and when to run. Defending my inability to do something is not a high priority early in the morning. I have learned that to maintain peace and order in the house, I have to bite my tongue.

Later on the same day, something happened which turned my cloudy day into a sunny one. Kindness always changes people's hearts.

I was in the waiting room of Dr. Kim Stock, my primary physician, who had ordered an ultrasound procedure for my heart because she had detected a slight heart murmur during my last physical checkup.

The young woman looking at my chart smiled, looked surprised and said, "Oh my! What is your secret? When I read the personal data that indicated you are an 86-year-old man, I was expecting to see an old man in a wheelchair, or at least with a cane. I thought I had the wrong patient."

"You are an angel sent by God. I had a bad day earlier," I told the young lab technician. Her kind and complimentary words were like drops of rain falling onto dry soil.

Isn't that amazing? I am always stunned at God's ways. Earlier, I felt sorry for myself because I am not muscular like Mark. But God lifted me up by sending to me a kind and sweet lab technician.

I thank and praise our Father, God, for giving me a relatively healthy and long life. In 1998, when I went home to the Philippines, I learned that only four of us were left from the 1951 sixth-grade class of Balilihan Central Elementary school, in the province of Bohol in the Philippines.

Think about it. My heart has been pumping blood for 86 years. It is still pumping regularly, I do not know for how many more years.

I did not major in physics at school. But in my humble calculation, the energy that my heart has put out for more than eight decades without failing probably could lift up the entire Empire State Building.

My heart is an amazing pump! Have you ever heard of any pump that functioned for 86 years regularly without an interruption?

The heart is God's awesome creation. Let's look at it from a different angle.

"There is a God-shaped vacuum in the heart of each man, which cannot be satisfied by any created thing but only by God the Creator, made known through Jesus Christ," said Blaise Pascal, who had one of the greatest minds in history.

"God has put eternity in man's heart," King Solomon said.

The eternity which is in man's heart is God's image. Though God's image in us is marred by sin, our heart yearns for something more than the world cans offer.

As a result, our rebellious heart continuously, even desperately, runs after things to fill the void in our heart that is reserved for God.

Saint Augustine writes in his *Confessions*, "**You have made us for yourself, O Lord, and our hearts are restless until they rest in You.**" Augustine's most often quoted phrase captures something that resonates deep within the human person.

The truth of the God-shaped vacuum in our heart brings me to the story of the woman at the well of Samaria who encountered Jesus.

She found her heart's rest there. She had been married to five men. Her life was a mess until she encountered Jesus.

On a particular day, she went to the well at noon. It is very hot at noon. People went to the well in morning. Why did she go to the well at noon? Maybe she needed extra water.

Or maybe she wanted to avoid the town's other women. Walking under the hot summer sun was a small price to pay to escape their sharp tongues.

She expected silence and solitude. Instead she found Jesus.

Jesus asked her for water. But she was too streetwise to think all Jesus wanted was a drink.

"Since when does a Jew like you ask a woman like me for water?" she asked. She wanted to know what Jesus really had in mind.

She was right; Jesus was interested in more than water. He was interested in her heart.

They talked. She could not remember the last time a man had spoken to her with respect. Jesus told her of a spring that would quench the thirst not of the throat, but of the soul.

That intrigued her. "Sir, give me this water so that I won't get thirsty and have to keep coming here to draw water," she said.

"Go tell your husband and come back," Jesus told her.

Her heart sank. Here was a man with a gentleness she never had seen before. Now he was asking her about her husband. Anything but that.

Maybe she considered lying or changing the subject. Perhaps she wanted to leave, but she stayed and told the truth.

"I have no husband," she said. Kindness has a way of inviting honesty.

The woman must have wondered what Jesus would do next or if Jesus' kindness would cease when the truth was revealed.

"Will he be angry?" or "Will he leave?" or "Will he think I am worthless?

If you have the same anxieties, pay attention.

"You are right. You have no husband. The man you are living with now is not your husband," Jesus said.

No criticism. No anger. No "what-kind-of mess-you-have-made-of-your-life" lecture. It was not perfection that Jesus was seeking; it was honesty.

The woman was amazed. "There is something different about you. Do you mind if I ask you something?" she said.

Then she asked a question that revealed a big hole in her soul: "Where is God? My people say He is on the mountain. Your people say He is in Jerusalem. I do not know where He is."

Can you imagine the expression on Jesus' face when He heard the question? Of all the places to find a hungry heart – Samaria; of all Samaritans searching for God – a woman; of all women hungry for God – a five-time divorcee.

Of all the people chosen to personally receive the secret of all the ages – an outcast among outcasts, the most insignificant person in town.

Jesus did not reveal the secret to Herod or to the Sanhedrin. It was not revealed in the colonnades of the Roman court that Jesus announced His identity.

No. Jesus revealed it in the shade of a well of a rejected land to an ostracized woman. Jesus' eyes must have danced as He whispered the secret: "I AM THE MESSIAH!"

CHAPTER 9

Jesus says,

"Come to Me"

The other day, my care receiver screamed at me as we were driving home from a beauty shop appointment. "I can no longer stand it to live at home! Your attitude stinks. You do not like to take care of me. I would be much better off in a nursing home. I am tired of looking at your negative face! Find me a nursing home," she said.

I thought to myself, "Go ahead, make my day! You would be doing me a big favor." But I did not respond. I wanted to avoid a "third world war."

"I was so angry at you at the beauty shop today. If I had a gun, I would have killed you," she said.

"What did I do that was so bad?" I gently inquired. All I did was ask Mark, her hair stylist, to cut my hair while we were waiting for her hair to dry.

"Why did you ask Mark to cut your hair at the same time I was having my hair done? You have no respect for me," she screamed.

I told her I was sorry, but my tone probably was more of sarcasm than surprise.

"You always say that you are sorry, but you never change," she replied. "You are like an old dog. You could never learn new tricks."

She is right. I am an old dog. My ways are set. But I am pretty comfortable with who I am. I am pretty much at peace with myself.

I didn't know that a woman's hair appointment is so sacred that whoever interferes with it might as well be in front of a death squad. I thought that if Mark cut my hair today, then I wouldn't have to leave my care receiver so I could get a haircut tomorrow. Leaving her alone at home always causes anxiety for both of us.

I thought I had a brilliant idea, but I was wrong.

Thanks to God, I did not lose my marbles. The whole episode did not make sense to me. The trigger point (interfering with a hair appointment) was not serious enough for her to want to leave home and go to a nursing home.

"My care receiver is having a temporary nervous breakdown," I thought to myself.

I was right. It was temporary. After a few minutes, my care receiver became her old self.

"If you no longer want to live at home and move to a nursing home, that is OK. We will find you a good one. But think hard before you make your decision," I told her. "Remember that the grass on the other side always looks greener."

"I know you are tired of seeing my old face 24/7," I continued. "In a nursing home, you will see many beautiful faces; you will encounter many sorts of personalities. Some of them will be good-natured and others will be nasty."

"But I guarantee you that the services you will get in a nursing home will not be as good as the services I give you at home. The people in the nursing are workers. The service I give you comes from a person who loves and cares for you."

Some events I encounter while caregiving get on my nerves. They siphon peace and energy from my hole being. But by the grace of God, every time I hit my lowest low, Jesus comes to the rescue.

To me, one of the most endearing phrases of Jesus is "**Come to me.**" What a beautiful thought – I am coming to Jesus!

This invitation reminds me of something that happened to me a long time ago when I had just arrived in the United States from the Philippines.

I accepted my friend's invitation, even I did not know where we were going. At that time, I was not familiar with the American culture. I knew what "happy" meant and I knew what "hour" meant. But I did not know the meaning of "happy hour".

My friends took me to a bar for a "happy hour." I had never heard that phrase before. "Holy hour," yes; I had been to many of them. But I had never been part of a "happy hour."

The bar was dimply lit; the conversations were loud; the cigarette smoke filled the place (smoking was not illegal at bars and restaurants at that time).

"This is a place where people unwind at the end of their working week," a friend told me. And unwind they did.

It is true that happy hour makes people forget their troubles. But more troubles come afterward; happy hour is a temporary fix. People often pay for it with a hangover the day after.

We all crave happiness and peace in our heart, but often we look for them in the wrong places.

God is like a magnet and our hearts are like pieces of iron. Whenever we seek goodness, happiness and peace, we are seeking God, Who is the ultimate goodness, the ultimate happiness and the ultimate peace.

Only Jesus can lead us to true happiness and peace – a happiness that does not last only for an hour, but is without end.

Jesus knows our burdens. He knows our guilt and our unconfessed sins, poor health, troubled marriages and frustrations in caregiving.

True peace and happiness can come only when we enter into a dialogue with the God Who is passionately in love with us, Who has sent His Son for us to destroy the power of sin and death, Who longs to share with us not only His gift of friendship, but also the gift of His life forever in heaven.

True peace and happiness cans come into our heart only when we commit ourselves to love our neighbors, share what we have with those in need and read God's word daily, where we can hear Him speak to us in the depths of our being, saying **"Come to Me and I will give you rest."**

CHAPTER 10

God felt our pains and experienced our fears

I started my day at Quick Lube to get an oil change for my Mazda and the technician told me I needed four tires. "You need to change your tires right away. They are all cracking and could explode at any time," he said.

I took a deep breath as dollar signs flashed through my mind.

While the technician was talking, my phone rang. My care receiver wanted me home immediately because she needed help to go the bathroom. "Oh, no. Not that again," I said to myself. The same thing often had occurred lately.

Unfortunately, I arrived too late and had to clean the mess which resulted – not a part of my day's plan.

Afterwards, I drove to my local tire store, only to find that it had closed and moved to another town.

Have you had a day like this? Jesus had many. This is one of the reasons why Jesus understands my bad days. Here is one example.

The day, started with bad news when a messenger told Jesus, "Your cousin John the Baptist is dead! King Herod had his head cut off!" Can you imagine Jesus' pain at hearing the news?

Then the messenger told Him, "We think Herod is after your head, too. Herod does not like the things he hears that you have been doing."

To take a break, Jesus decided to go with His disciples to a quiet place where they could rest and reflect. They took a boat to the other side of the lake where they were, away from the people who were following them.

Jesus needed to be alone for a few hours for a respite, a retreat, a time to pray. "The people can wait till tomorrow," He thought.

But the people had other ideas. They learned about Jesus' plan and walked six miles around the lake to meet Him on the other side. "Surprise!" they shouted.

The silent environment that Jesus had sought became as loud as Ohio Stadium on the Saturday of an Ohio State home game.

Jesus' plans were interrupted. What He had in mind for His day and what the people had in mind were two different agendas. What Jesus sought and what Jesus got were not the same.

Jesus knows how I feel on difficult days. Like mine, Jesus' pulse has raced; His eyes have grown weary; His heart has grown heavy; He has climbed out of bed with a sore throat; He has been kept awake late and gotten up early. He can relate to the hustle and bustle of my daily life.

"For we have no superhuman High Priest to whom our weaknesses are unintelligible. He Himself shared fully in all our experiences and temptation, except that He never sinned" (Hebrews 4:15).

St. Paul boldly proclaims Jesus' ability to understand how we feel. Look at the wording again.

He Himself: Not an angel, not an ambassador, not a messenger but Jesus Himeslf.

Shared fully: not partially, not nearly, not to a large degree, but entirely. Jesus shared fully.

In all our experience: every hurt, every ache, all the stresses and the strains. No exceptions, no substitutes. Why? So Jesus could sympathize with our weaknesses.

He did this for the same reason a politician wears a hard hat and enters a factory to identify with the employees, a social worker spends the night in the street among homeless people or a general eats in the mess hall with the enlisted men.

"I identify with you; I can understand; I can relate." All three instances are an attempt to communicate the same message.

But the factory employees know the politician will leave when the TV crew is gone; the homeless people know the social worker will be in a warm bed tomorrow night; the soldiers know the general will be eating in the officers' quarters after the visit.

For, these professionals, their participation is partial. But Jesus' participation in our humanity was complete. Jesus shared fully in all our experiences.

Every page of the Gospel hammers home this crucial principle: **God knows how you feel.**

When you tell God that you have reached your limit, God knows what you mean. God knows it, too, when you shake your head at impossible deadlines.

When your plans are interrupted by people who have other plans, God nods in empathy. God has been there. He knows how you feel.

Here is an example to illustrate how amazing it is that God became human to share our pain:

It happened on Feb. 15, 1921 in the operating room of Kane Summit Hospital in New York City. A doctor was performing an appendectomy.

The events leading to the surgery were uneventful; the patient complained of a severe abdominal pain and the diagnosis was clear – an inflamed appendix.

Dr. Evan O'Neill Kane was in charge of the surgery. In his distinguished 37-year medical career, he had performed nearly 4,000 appendectomies, so this surgery was uneventful in all ways, except two.

The first: Local anesthesia was being used in a major surgery for the first time in history. Dr. Kane was a crusader against the hazards of general anesthesia. He contended that local anesthesia was far safer.

Many of his colleagues agreed with him in principal. But for them to agree in practice, they would have to see the theory applied.

Dr. Kane searched for a volunteer, a patient who was willing to undergo surgery while under local anesthesia. A volunteer was not easy to find.

Many people were squeamish at the thought of being awake during their own surgery. Others were worried that the anesthesia might wear off too soon.

But eventually, Dr. Kane found a candidate and on Tuesday morning, Feb. 15, the historic surgery occurred.

The patient was prepared and wheeled to the operating room. Local anesthesia was applied. As Dr. Kane had done thousands of times, he dissected the superficial tissue and located the appendix. He skillfully removed it and concluded the surgery. During the procedure, the patient complained only of minor discomfort.

The volunteer was taken into post-op, placed in his hospital room, recovered quickly and was released two days later.

Dr. Kane had proven his theory. Thanks to the willingness of a brave volunteer, he had demonstrated that local anesthesia is a viable and even a preferable alternative.

I said that two things made the surgery unique. You know the first: it was the use of local anesthesia for the first time in a major operation.

The second thing that was special was the patient's identity. The courageous candidate for Dr. Kane was – Dr. Kane!

To prove his point, Dr. Kane had operated on himself. The doctor became a patient so he convince patients to trust the doctor (From Paul Harvey's *The Rest of the Story*).

"That is hard to believe!" many people may say.

And it is! But the story of a doctor who became his own patient is mild compared to the story of a God who became human. Jesus did that.

Why did Jesus do it?

So that you and I would believe that the Healer knows our hurts, He voluntarily became one of us. God placed Himself in our position. He suffered our pains and felt our fears.

Rejection? God felt it. Temptation? God knew it. Loneliness? God experienced it. Death? God tasted it, so that when you hurt, you can go to him – your Father and your Physician – and let Him heal you.

CHAPTER 11

Jesus paid a great price to take you home

Caregiving is a choice. I know that my care is not perfect, but I do my best. I need to forgive myself when I lose my temper and to try again tomorrow.

Thinking that Jesus understands what I am going through helps me to be more compassionate with my care receiver.

When Jesus and His disciples landed on the other side of the lake, a huge crowd was waiting. He had compassion on the people and healed the sick.

I doubt if anyone in the crowd thought of asking Jesus how He was doing. There was never an indication that anyone in the crowds following Him was ever interested in knowing how Jesus was feeling. It seems no one came to give to Him; all came to take.

When hands were extended and voices demanded something from Him, Jesus responded with love.

"Jesus healed the sick." Matthew wrote. Not just some of the sick or only the righteous among the sick.

Since Jesus knew the secrets of people's hearts, I wonder if Jesus was tempted to say to a rapist, "Heal you after what you have done?" Or to a child molester, "Why should I heal you?" Or to a bigot, "Get out of here and take your arrogance with you."

Why do I wonder about this? Because Jesus could see our past and our future. Unfortunately, I'm sure there were some among those He healed who would hurt others in the future. He may have released tongues that would curse, given sight to those who would lust, or healed hands that would kill.

Not many of those Jesus healed said "Thank you," but he healed them anyway. Most of them would be more concerned about being healthy than being holy. But he healed them anyway. Some of those who cried for bread on one day would cry for his blood months later. But he healed them anyway.

Jesus gave gifts to people knowing full well that those gifts could be used for evil.

For everyone Jesus healed, He had to overlook the future and the past. He still does.

God does not ask you to prove that you will put your salary to good use, nor does He turn off your oxygen supply when you misuse His gifts, nor does He give you only the gifts you thank Him for.

God gives gifts because of His nature and not because of our worthiness.

On the day of the miracle of the loaves and fishes, Jesus was not stressed out, but his disciples were. "Send the people away!" they told Jesus.

"After all, you have taught them. You healed them. You have accommodated them. And now if you do not send them away, they will ask you to feed them, too," the disciples thought to themselves.

"They do not need to go away. Give them something to eat," Jesus told His disciples. I wish I could have seen the look on their faces when they heard what Jesus said.

The disciples, instead of looking at God, looked at their wallets.

"The amount we need to feed the crowd is equivalent to eight months' salary for a man. Are we going to spend that much on bread so that everyone could eat?" they thought.

Other thoughts may have been "Jesus, you have got to be kidding!" Or "Jesus, you can't be serious." Or "Jesus, is this one of your jokes?" Or "For heaven's sake, Jesus, do you know how many people are there?"

While Jesus saw the crowd as an opportunity to love, the disciples saw the crowd as a problem.

It was as if the disciples were telling the ***Bread of Life*** that there was no bread. How silly that must have appeared.

At this point, Jesus could have given up. His disciples could not do what He was asking them to do. In front of 5,000 men, plus women and children, His disciples let Him down.

But instead of rebuking them, Jesus asked "How many loaves do you have?"

The disciples brought a little boy's lunch. The lunch pail provided enough for a banquet and all were fed without a reprimand, a word of anger; or an "I told you so" from Jesus. He had the same compassion for the crowd as

He had for his disciples.

To emphasize the point that Jesus understands how we feel, I would like to retell a story I heard a long time ago.

A little boy was looking for a puppy. He went to a pet shop. The owner showed him a litter of puppies in a box. The boy picked each one up, examined them and put them back in the box.

Then he went to the owner and said, "I picked one out. How much will it cost?"

The owner told the boy the price. The boy promised to come back soon with the money. "Do not wait too long," the owner cautioned. "Puppies like these sell quickly."

The boy turned, smiled and confidentially told the owner, "I am not worried. Mine will still be here."

The boy went to work weeding, washing windows and cleaning yards. He worked hard and saved his money. When he had enough to purchase the puppy, he returned to the pet store.

The boy walked to the counter and laid the money down. The owner counted the cash, verified the amount, smiled and told the boy, "All right son, you can get your puppy."

The boy reached into the back of the box, pulled out a skinny puppy with a limp leg and started to leave.

The owner stopped the boy. "Don't take that puppy," the owner objected. "He is crippled. He can't play. He will never run with you. He can't fetch. Get one of the healthy pups."

"No thank you, sir," the boy replied. "This is exactly the dog I am looking for".

As the boy started to leave, the owner started to speak but remained silent. Suddenly the owner understood. Extending from the boy's pants was a brace – a brace for his crippled leg.

The boy knew how the puppy felt. He knew the puppy was very special.

Jesus knows how you feel. You are under the gun at work, He knows how you feel. You have got to do more than humanly possible. He knows how you feel.

You are precious to Jesus, so precious that He became like you so you would come to Him.

When you struggle, Jesus knows how you feel. When you yearn, Jesus responds. When you ask questions, Jesus listens. Jesus has been there.

Remember, my friend, that Jesus loves you, period. His love for you is unconditional. Jesus does not love you more when you are being good. Jesus does not love you less when you are not being good. Jesus loves you, period.

Jesus is like the crippled boy and you are like the crippled puppy. You are special to Jesus.

Like the crippled boy, Jesus paid a great price to take you home to the Father.

God sees with a Father's eyes; He sees our defects and blemishes. But He also sees our value. In God's eyes, every human being is a treasure. In God's eyes, people are not a source of stress, they are a source of joy.

CHAPTER 12

God's peace surpasses all understanding

Almost every time I step out of the house, my care receiver anxiously says, "I am always afraid every time you leave. What if you have an accident and you do not come back. "Who will take care of me?" Or " If you have a heart attack I do not know what I would do."

Too many "if's" could be a sign of an anxiety disorder.

"God will take care of you" is my menta; This is my response to those questions. But I never verbalize it. Verbalizing it would sound too callous or uncaring.

I have assured my care receiver that I have made arrangements where she would go if something happens to me. You have a place to g, if I can no longer take care of you."

Deep in my heart, I know that God's providence will take care of all of us, like He takes care of the birds in the air and the flowers in the meadows. God knows of every single hair that drops to the ground. We are precious to God. We are His children.

Nothing happens to us without God's knowing it or without God's allowing it to happen.

My care receiver's concern is a valid one. But her concerns should not make her life a hostage to anxiety. That is not God's will for us.

Do you sometimes experience anxiety attacks? Or do you know someone who does?

Do you know that according to the National Institute of Mental Health, anxiety disorders are reaching epidemic proportions?

Researchers say that in a given year, nearly 50 million Americans will feel the effects of panic attacks, phobias or other anxiety disorders.

According to the Journal of American Medical Association, people of each generation in the 20th century were three times more likely to experience depression than people of the preceding generation.

Stress-related ailments cost the nation $399 billion every year in medical bills and loss of productivity, while our use of sedative drugs keeps skyrocketing.

"Do not fret," the psalmist wrote, "it only causes harm." Yes, it does. It causes harm to our necks, our jaws, our backs and our voice.

Anxiety can make our eyes twitch, blood pressure rise, heads ache and armpits sweat. Anxiety isn't fun.

Congratulations to us Americans. The United States is now the most anxious country in the world. The land of stars and stripes has become a country of stress and strife.

You may ask, "What's going on?" Our cars are safer than ever. Citizens are more educated. Food, water and electricity are regulated. Though gangs exist in our cities, Americans do not live under the danger of imminent attack.

Citizens in Third Wrld countries, despite having fewer of the basic life necessities, enjoy more tranquility than we Americans do.

When these less anxious developing-world citizens immigrate to the United States, they tend to get just as anxious as Americans. There is something in the American way of life that make people anxious.

What makes citizens in our culture so anxious? Researchers think that one reason for increased anxiety is the rapid change in our society.

In our parents' generation, an earthquake in Morocco would be reported on the evening newscast. In our generation, the event is reported in minutes and repeated over and over during the day.

"We move faster than before," researchers say.

Our ancestors traveled as far as a horse or a camel could travel during daylight. Not us. We jet through time zones as if they were neighborhood streets.

When the sun sets, our ancestors turned off their brains.

Not us. We turn on cable news; we open our laptopss; we look at our computers or phone screens. We fall asleep with accounts of murders and catastrophes fresh in our brain.

On a more personal level, most of us know people who are facing foreclosure, fighting cancer, slogging through divorce or battling addiction. You or someone you know is bankrupt, broke or going out of business.

One would think that we Christians are exempt from worry, but we are not. Despite what we have been taught, a Christian life is not a life of peace.

When we do not have peace, we assume that the problem is within us. Not only do we feel anxious, we also feel guilty about our anxiety. It is like a downward spiral of anxiety, guilt and more anxiety.

And here comes St. Paul saying: "Be anxious for nothing" (Philippians 4:6).h

"What in the heck Paul is saying? Is Paul out of touch?" I ask myself. Paul does not say "Be anxious a little." This would have been enough. Or "Be anxious only when things are really bad." No, he did no say that. Instead, he said, "Be anxious for nothing."

When we take a deeper look at what Paul is saying, we realize he is telling us, "Do not live in perpetual anxiety. In life, anxiety is unavoidable. Butalways living in a state of anxiety is a choice."

Jesus warns us, "Be careful or your hearts will be weighed down with ... anxieties of life" (Luke 21:34).

Is your heart weighed down with worry? If it is, Scripture has this to say.

"Rejoice in the Lord always. Again, I will say rejoice! Let your gentleness be known to men. The Lord is at hand. Be anxious for nothing, but in everything, by prayer and supplication, with thanksgiving let your request be known to

God; and the peace of God, which surpasses all understanding, will guard your hearts and minds through Christ Jesus. Finally, brethren, whatever things are true, whatever things are noble, whatever things are just, whatever things are pure, whatever things are lovely, whatever things are of good report, if there is any virtue and if there anything praiseworthy – meditate on these things" (Philippians 4: 4-8).

The peace of God, which surpasses all understanding, will *guard your hearts and minds!* What a beautiful promise!

Rejoice in the Lord always; Let us celebrate God's goodness. Take a vacation from your phone or laptop and slow down to smell the roses. Enjoy the beautiful sunsets and sunrises.

Let your request be known to God; Let us always ask for God's help. Though the world seems to be out of control, know that God is in control. Make God the center of every decision you make.

…with thanksgiving: Before you lay down to rest every night, kneel and give thanks to the Lord for all the things He has done for you during the day. Give God the glory for the good things you have done; ask forgiveness for your failures and strive to do better tomorrow.

Let us leave our concerns with God and let us meditate on the things that are good and worthy of praise.

Living a life of perpetual anxiety is not the will of God for us. Facing dread and trepidation every day is not the will of God for us.

Jesus spoke to storms. He will speak to ours. Jesus calmed the hearts of the apostles. He will calm ours. Jesus told the Apostles not to fear. Jesus is telling us the same.

With God's grace, we will be anxious for nothing and discover God's peace – the peace that surpasses all understanding.

CHAPTER 13

Fill your mind with thoughts of God

Being a caregiver is like being hit by a Category-5 hurricane. A caregiver needs a strong foundation to survive in the storm.

Strong hurricanes have been hitting the United States lately. Some say these storms are getting stronger and bigger because of global warming. Fortunately, in America the warning systems are pretty much efficient and accurate, and there are shelters where people can go to protect themselves from flood and strong winds.

Have you ever been caught in a storm of life?

Sadly, those types of storms are not limited to strong winds and severe flooding. Sometimes storms can come to us in three big D's: difficulties, divorce and death.

Do you know where to seek shelter from those storms?

St. Paul did. If anyone had reasons to be anxious, Paul had. When Paul was about 60 years old, he found himself in a Roman prison (I saw the prison when I attended a meeting of diocesan mission directors in Rome).

When Paul was in prison, he had been a Christian for 30 years. His back was badly bent because of his extensive travels to many places to spread the Gospel.

The many beatings he endured as a Christian contributed to his back problems. Paul received 39 lashes on five different occasions; he was beaten with rods on three. Once he was left for dead.

He had been imprisoned and deserted by friends and co-workers and had endured shipwrecks, storms and starvation.

He was half-blind. What's more, he was awaiting trial before the Roman emperor. Nero was best-known for killing Christians and Paul was the best-known Christian at that time.

If you were not familiar with Paul's difficult life and his gloomy future, you would think when you read his letter to the Philippians that he was vacationing in a hotel in the Bahamas, enjoying a sunny beach with a martini in his hand.

His letter did not contain a word of fear or complaint. He never shook his fist at God. Instead, Paul gave thanks to God and asked his readers to do the same.

"Rejoice in the Lord always. Again, I say rejoice!" (Philippians 4:4). How can a person obey such a command? Is it possible for a person to be in a constant state of gladness without interruption?

Of course, the answer to the question is "No." It is not possible to be in such a state. But that was not what Paul meant by *"Rejoice in the Lord always."*

What he meant was to remain in the Lord even when storms are raging around you.

Paul is not talking about feelings. Rather, what he is saying was a call to make a conscious decision to stay in the Lord, a decision deeply rooted in the belief that God exists, that God is in control and that God is good.

Paul held firm to this belief. This belief is in the center of his soul. Let Nero rage and let storms rage. Paul's faith would never collapse. His faith was established in a strong belief system.

How strong is your belief system? Your beliefs are your answer to the fundamental questions about life, such as "Is anyone in control of the universe?" Or "Does life have a purpose?" Or "Do I have value?" Or "Is this life all there is?"

Your belief system has nothing to do with the color of your skin, your appearance, your talents or your age. Your belief system has nothing to do with the exterior. Rather, it is more of the interior. It is a set of convictions, all unseen, upon which your faith depends.

If your belief system is strong, you will withstand the storms of life. If it is weak, the storms will prevail.

If you want to change a person's response to life, change what the person believes about life. Your belief system is the most important thing about you.

A strong belief system in anchored in the sovereignty of God, in the belief that God is in perfect control of the universe; that He preserves and governs every element in the universe; that He is directly involved with all created things, directing them to act in a way that fulfills his divine purpose.

Most stressed people are control freaks. The more they try to control the world, the more they realize that they cannot.

Scripture has a better idea. Rather than seek control, relinquish control. You cannot run the world. But you can entrust the world to God.

This is the message behind Paul's admonition to "*rejoice in the Lord.*" Peace is within reach, not for lack of problems but because of the presence of the sovereign Lord.

Rather than be upset by the chaos of the world, rejoice in the Lord's sovereignty as Paul did.

"*The things which happened to me had actually turned out for the furtherance of the Gospel, so that it has become evident to the whole palace guard, and to all the rest that my chains are in Christ*" (Philippians 1: 12-13), Paul said.

To read Paul's letter to the Philippians is to read the words of a man who in the innermost part of his being believes in the steady hand of a good God.

To survive in the storms of life, you need to anchor your soul in the sovereignty of God Who reigns supreme over every detail of the universe.

What is God's answer to our troubled times? Heaven has an occupied throne. God is in charge.

Do not approach your problems with wringing hands; rather, approach them with bended knees.

The next time you fear the future, rejoice in the Lord's sovereignty. Rejoice in what He has accomplished. Rejoice that God is able to do what you cannot do. Fill your mind with the thought of God.

The mind cannot be full of God and full of fear at the same time. Trust in this: *"He* (God) *will keep in perfect peace all those who trust in him, whose thoughts turn often to the Lord"* (Isaiah 26:3).

Do not get lost in your troubles. Believe that good things will happen. Trust in what God is saying to you: *"In everything God works for the good of those who love him"* (Romans 8:28).

Your firm belief in God's sovereignty will melt away your anxieties like ice on a July sidewalk.

CHAPTER 14

I trust in God's mercy

As a caregiver, sometimes I am a nervous wreck. I also feel like I am on a one-way street, always giving but never receiving in return. When I get a "thank you" from my care receiver, I am very grateful because they are slow in coming.

I know I am becoming a grumpy old man. That feeling makes me anxious and my anxiety makes me feel guilty. I feel I am on a downward spiral of anxiety and guilt.

Thanks be to God that when I find myself in a place where dark is darker, He showers me with flickers of light which allow me to see things from a different angle – the angle of his love and mercy.

Have you ever wondered how anxiety and guilt found their way into our world?

This is how Scripture answers the question: *"That evening, Adam and Eve heard the sound of the Lord God walking in the garden; and they hid themselves from among the trees"* (Genesis 3:8).

What happened to the first family? Until that point, there was no trepidation. They did not feel any fear. They had never hidden from God. Indeed, they had nothing to hide *"Adam and Eve were naked, but they felt no shame"* (Genesis 2:25).

Then came the snake and the forbidden fruit. Adam and Eve said "Yes" to the snake and said "No" to God. And when they did, their lives collapsed like an accordion. They went into hiding, feeling ashamed.

Guilt came first and anxiety came next. Adam and Eve did not know how to process their failure. Neither do we.

Unresolved guilt could turn into a frightful mess. After his affair with Bathsheba, David wrote: *"When I refused to confess my sin, my body wasted away and I groaned all day long. Day and night your hand of discipline was heavy on me. My strength evaporated like water in the summer heat"* (Psalm 32: 3-4).

Guilt sucks the life from our soul. Grace restores it.

I learned from Paul. He clung to grace and relied on the mercy of God.

Paul had every reason to feel guilty. He orchestrated the death of Christians. He was a terrorist in his time. He took believers into custody. He spilled the blood of Christians.

"Paul was like a wild man going everywhere to devastate believers, even entering private homes and dragging men and women alike and jailing them" (Acts 8:3), Peter said.

Paul had blood on his hands. But something happened to Paul on the road to Damascus. Jesus appeared to him. Once he encountered Jesus, he could see no more. He could not see any other option except to spend the rest of his life talking less about himself and more about Jesus.

"But all these things that I thought worthwhile – now I have thrown them all away so that I can put my trust and hope in Christ alone" (Philippians 3:7), Paul said.

Paul gave his guilt to Jesus. He surrendered his guilt to Jesus.

"I am still not all I should be, but I am bringing all my energies to bear on this one thing: Forgetting the past and looking forward to what lies ahead, I strain to reach the end of the race and receive the prize for which God is calling us up to heaven because of what Jesus did for us" (Philippians 3: 13–14). Paul said.

Are you burdened with guilt? If you are, do what Paul did. Go to God and rejoice in His mercy. Trust in God's ability to forgive. Cast yourself upon the grace of Christ and Christ alone.

Do not wallow in the mud of your guilt. Give it to Jesus. Your future matters more than your past. That is why a windshield is bigger than a rearview mirror.

God's grace is greater than your sin. What you did was not good, but your God is good. And God will forgive you. He is ready to write a new chapter of your life.

I have learned from Paul's life that to be at peace is to recognize the severity of sin and the immensity of grace; to dwell on grace and not on guilt.

Think about it. Someday we all will stand before God. All of us will be present; all of us will give an account for our lives – every thought, every word, every action. This event would be terrifying without God's grace.

Thanks to God for sending Jesus to earth to take away the sins of the world (John 1:29). On judgement day, when the list of my sins will appear, I can turn to Jesus and will say to Him, "Lord, you took my sins away."

In one of Henri Nouwen's books, he tells about the lesson of trust he learned from a family of trapeze artists known as the Flying Rodleighs. He visited with them for a time after watching them fly through the air with elegant poise. When he asked one of the flyers the secret of trapeze artists, the acrobat gave this reply:

"The secret is that the flyer does nothing and the catcher does everything. When I fly to Joe (the catcher,) I have simply to stretch out my arms and hands and wait for him to catch me and pull me safely to a platform.

The worst thing the flyer can do is to try to catch the catcher. I am not supposed to catch Joe. It is Joe's task to catch me. If I grab Joe's wrists, I might break them or might break mine, and that would be the end for both of us. A flyer must fly and a catcher must catch and the flyer must trust outreached arms will be there for him."

The act of salvation is like a trapeze. God is the catcher and we are the flyers. We trust; we rely solely on God's ability to catch us. As we do, a wonderful thing happens – we fly elegantly.

God our Father has not dropped anyone. He will not drop you. His grip is steady and His hands are open.

May God grant us grace to proclaim, like Paul: "*I know the Lord will continue to rescue me from every trip, trap, snare and pitfall of evil and carry me safely to his heavenly kingdom. May He be glorified throughout eternity*" (2 Timothy 4:18).

Place yourself in God's loving care. As you do, God's peace will flood your soul. You will learn to rejoice in the Lord always.

CHAPTER 15

Don't let anxiety stalk you every day of your life

It is difficult to watch your loved one suffer. Imagine how you would feel if you completely depended on someone to help transfer you from your bed to a wheelchair and to help you position yourself on the toilet seat?

What if you could not go on your own to the fridge to get a snack? I cannot imagine how frustrating that situation would be.

Caregiving and care receiving are both difficult. Thanks to God for His graces that help us carry our daily burdens.

In spite of the pressures of life, Scripture urges us to rejoice. "*Rejoice in the Lord always*" (Phil. 4:4), Paul tells us. Not only when things go well, not only on weekends, not only on Christmas, not only when you receive a promotion, not only on your birthday, but *always*.

But how can Mary, my dear friend who is battling cancer, rejoice always? Or my neighbor Joe who received a pink slip yesterday? Or Jane, who has delivered a baby with a disability? Or my care receiver, who is bedridden?

To rejoice when things are good sounds normal. But to rejoice when things are bad sounds corny.

But Paul and Joseph rejoiced in the midst of horrible situations – Paul in a Roman prison and Joseph in an Egyptian dungeon.

Joseph's jail was dank and dark, an underground dungeon with windowless rooms, stale food and bitter water. He had no way out.

Joseph's troubles started with his brothers not liking his dreams and deciding to kill him by throwing him into a pit. Joseph would have been dead had their brothers' thirst for blood been stronger than their greed.

When the opportunity arose, instead of killing Joseph, they sold him to traveling merchants bound for Egypt.

In Egypt, Joseph was auctioned like an animal and sold to the highest bidder – Pharoah.

While working at Pharaoh's household, his wife desired Joseph. She seduced him and he ran away, leaving her holding his coat. Then she accused Joseph of attempted rape. Pharoah took his wife's side. Joseph landed in jail for a crime he did not commit.

In prison, Joseph was a model prisoner. The warden was impressed with Joseph's behavior and made him the "convict-in-charge."

Joseph languished in the prison for two years without any hope of being released.

I wonder if, during his incarceration, Joseph ever asked questions like "Is this the way God treats his children?" Or "Is this God's reward for good behavior?" Or "You do your best, and this is what you get – a jail cell and a hard bed?" Or "Why me, Lord?"

We do not know if Joseph asked these questions. But we too face adversities in life, such as loss of a loved one, dealing with cancer or a broken relationship or financial difficulties. These may leave us wondering, "Is there a God?"

Of course there is a God. Our God is personally and powerfully involved in His creation.

Scripture says *"The Son is the radiance of God's glory and the exact presentation of his being, sustaining all things by his powerful word"* (Hebrews 1:3).

Jesus is directing the whole of creation toward God's desired end. Jesus is continually active in God's creation. Jesus exercises primacy over all things. *"He is before all things, and in him things are held together"* (Colossians 1:17).

Were Jesus to step back, the whole of creation would collapse. Without Jesus, all of creation would evaporate. Scripture says *"For in Him we live and move and have our being"* (Acts 17:28).

God is the one *"who causes the sun to rise on the evil and the good and sends his rain on the righteous and on the unrighteous"* (Matthew 5:45).

God is the one in charge of everything, even the details of our lives.

If God was in charge, why was Joseph in prison? Why is my friend's marriage in disarray? Why does God permit bad things to happen to us? Can God prevent bad things from happening to us?

Of course God can. Nothing happens to us without God knowing it or allowing it. God could turn our bad situations into blessings.

Look at what happened to Joseph. One minute he was in an Egyptian dungeon and the next minute he was the second-highest authority in Egypt.

This is how Joseph's situation changed from bad to good.

One night while Joseph was in prison, Pharaoh had a dream in which he saw seven thin cows eat seven fat cows. Pharaoh was deeply troubled by his dream. No one in Egypt could explain its meaning.

Someone told Pharaoh that there was someone in prison named Joseph who could interpret dreams, so Joseph was taken to Pharaoh.

"For seven years, there will be good harvests; after seven years, there will be worldwide famine." Joseph told Pharaoh.

"What shall we do?" Pharaoh asked Joseph.

"This is what you should do." Joseph said. "Build storage rooms and store as much grain as you can during the seven years of good harvest."

Pharaoh was impressed with Joseph's idea and turned to his cabinet members and said, "Gentlemen, I am putting Joseph in charge of preparing for the coming famine. He will answer to nobody except me."

When the famine came, Joseph's brothers from the land of Canaan went to Egypt to buy grain for their families.

Joseph's brothers did not recognize him, but Joseph recognized them. Their stomachs were bigger now and they had less hair. The last time Joseph saw them was when they were negotiating his price when he was sold to the merchants.

The tables had turned. Joseph now was on the top of the world, the No.2 man in Egypt. With a snap of his fingers, his brothers could turn into deviled eggs.

Revenge was in Joseph's hands. He could have punished his brothers for what they did to him. He had every reason to do this, but he did not.

Can you imagine the looks on the faces of Joseph's brothers when he revealed his identity to them?

In spite of his brothers' cruelty, Joseph was kind to them.

"You intended to harm me, but God intended it for good to accomplish, what is now being done, the saving of many lives. So do not be afraid. I will provide for you and your children" (Genesis 50:20 -21), Joseph assured his brothers.

Joseph viewed the sufferings of his life through the lens of divine providence.

May God grant us grace to do the same; otherwise, anxiety will stalk you every day of your life.

CHAPTER 16

Let your gentleness be evident to all

The past few days were very rough in our household. My wife (care receiver) fell from bed and hit her head at the edge of the bed table. As a result, she had a cut on her eyebrow which required a couple of stiches, her left shoulder socket was dislocated and her left arm was fractured.

I told the medical squad to take her to the Riverside Hospital emergency unit. Instead of riding with her in the ambulance, I was going to drive myself and meet them at the hospital.

I arrived at the hospital at 2 a.m. The folks at the emergency unit did not allow me to join my wife until she was assigned to a room.

I begged them to let me join her right away because she was incoherent. But they did not badge.

The emergency waiting room was full of people. One by one, they were called to join their loved ones. Every 10 minutes, I checked my wife's status.

At 4 a.m. I was the only one left in the waiting room. A nurse then told me, "Your wife is not in this hospital."

It was if my soul left my body. I had been waiting for almost five hours to join my wife and she was not in this hospital? Where was she? I began to wonder where the squad took my wife. I started to doubt that she had been taken to another hospital.

I was getting anxious. My wife had been on her own for almost five hours and was incoherent for all that time because of the fall.

"Could you call the squad to inquire where they took my wife?" I begged the nurse.

"No, we don't do that," the nurse responded. By that time, I felt I was going to have an anxiety attack.

"Let me go back to my computer and do some research," she said.

After a few minutes, she told me, "A few hours earlier, I saw your wife's name, but it is no longer on the admissions list."

What the nurse said dispelled some of my anxious feelings. "If the nurse saw her name on the computer several hours earlier, then my wife is in this hospital," I thought.

Eventually the nurse found my wife's room and I was escorted to join her.

It was a sad sight and a pitiful situation. She wore a neck brace and a sling to keep her dislocated arm in the shoulder socket and to keep it from moving.

She was delirious. She did not recognize me. She thought that I was the head of the Mafia trying to get her and put her away.

She became violent. I had to physically restrain her. She wanted to free herself from the vital-sign monitors and from the neck brace and sling.

She needed tough love from me. I am not good at it. My heart is too soft to do tough love. But at times, we have to do what we need to do.

There are times we have to step out from being gentle, for good reason. But God's command to be gentle must always be our mindset.

"Let your gentleness be evident to all. The Lord is near. Do not be anxious about anything" (Philippians 4: 5–6).

A gentle person is sober-minded, clear-thinking and contagiously calm.

Where can we get this gentleness? How can we keep our tempers from exploding? How can we keep our heads while others are losing theirs?

"The Lord is near." This is how the Scriptures answer the question.

You are not alone. You may feel alone. You may think you are alone. But there is never a moment when you face life without help. God is near.

In the Scriptures, God repeatedly pledges to us His loving presence.

"Do not be afraid. I am your shield, your exceedingly great reward" (Genesis 5:1), God said to Abraham.

"*Do not be afraid; God has heard*" (Genesis 21:17), an angel told Hagar.

"*Do not be afraid, for I am with you*" (Genesis 26:24), God reminded Isaac when Isaac was expelled from his land by the Philistines and forced to move from place to place.

"*Do not be afraid; do not be discouraged for the Lord your God will be with you wherever you go*" (Joshua 1:9), God told Joshua after Moses died.

God was with David in spite of his adultery; with Jacob in spite of his conniving, with Elijah in spite of his lack of faith.

Jesus called himself "Emmanuel," which means "God with us." In Jesus, God became flesh like us. God defeated death. He remains with us in our hearts and in the Blessed Sacrament.

God is not watching you from a distance. God has not left you. Face your problems with God beside you. Always clutch the presence God with both hands and say, "*The Lord is with me; I will not be afraid. What can mere mortals do to me?*" (Psalm 118:6).

Paul's point is this: *Because the Lord is near, we need be anxious for nothing.*

We can calmly take our problems to the Lord because he is as near to us as our next breath.

This is the lesson in the miracle of the bread and fishes. The miracle of the bread is Jesus' approach to anxious hearts – Jesus asked them to do the impossible; Jesus told the Apostles to feed 5,000 men, plus women and children.

The Apostles wanted to get rid of everyone. They told Jesus, *"Send them away that they may go into the village to buy their own lunch"* (Matthew 14:15).

The Apostles had every reason to be anxious because they did not think enough about what they had witnessed Jesus doing in the past – healing the sick people, raising a dead girl, calming the angry waves.

The business of getting ride of our anxieties is like pulling stumps out of the ground. Some of your worries have deep root systems. Extracting them is hard work. It could be the toughest challenge in your life. But you do not have to do it alone.

Present the challenge to your Father and ask Him to help you. He will solve the issue.

Will He solve it immediately? Maybe. Or perhaps He wants you to learn patience.

This is for sure: Contagious calm will occur to the degree that you turn to Him.

CHAPTER 17

God loves to hear the sound of our voices

My wife fell from bed and her head hit a corner edge of a bed table. She fractured her left arm, was at Riverside Hospital for a week, then was transferred to the Grand Dublin rehabilitation facility.

The days she spent in both places were very stressful for both of us. She could not stand on her own, could not walk and, with a broken left arm, needed help to eat and to go to the bathroom.

She was told to "Push the red button if you need help" from a nurse. But the response to the call for help was very slow and at times, there were no response at all.

As a result, I had to be at the hospital and the rehab facility most of the time to help her out. Without my help, she could hardly eat her meals and sometimes had to stay in bed wet for hours.

There were many wonderful nurses and medical assistants, but some were nasty and mean to my wife. Both facilities were understaffed. "After the pandemic, workers in the medical profession became difficult to find," a rehab facility administrator told me.

Caregiving is a very difficult assignment from God. Many times, I have been tempted to give up, but every time I do, God always come to my rescue. He sends me flickers of light to shine in my darkness. He reminds me of His promises and makes me feel His presence.

In times when I feel helpless and hopeless, I am always reminded that when Jesus came into the world, He revealed to us that God is our Father. This revelation, along with God's graces, gives me strength to carry on.

We call God "Father" because this is what Jesus wants us to do. We touch God's heart when we call Him Father.

As God's children, we can turn to Him at every moment.

When we call, He answers us; He never delays; He does not put us on hold; He never tells you to call later. God loves the sound of our voices.

"Be anxious for nothing, but in everything, by prayer and supplication, with thanksgiving, let your request be known to God" (Philippians 4:16), Scripture tells us.

When we learn to leave our troubles in the hands of God, we eventually see God's hands in everything. Instead of despairing, we make our requests known to God.

In Scripture, we read about people who asked Jesus for help with their problems. In many cases, Jesus asked them, "What do you want me to do for you?" (Luke 18:41).

Why did Jesus ask? It was obvious to everyone on the scene that the blind man wanted to see again.

Jesus asked because He wanted the man to articulate his problem. Jesus wanted the man to be specific.

Jesus wants the same from us. He wants us to be specific in our prayers. *"Let your request be known to God."*

"Rabbi, let me recover my sight," the blind man asked.

And Jesus said to him, *"Go your way; your faith has made you well"* (Mark 10: 51–52) and immediately he recovered his sight and followed Jesus.

At the wedding at Cana, when Mary saw that the wine supply was getting low, she was specific, telling Her Son, *"They have no more wine"* (John 2:3).

In one of Jesus' parables, a needy man did not say *"Give me something to eat"*; rather, he was specific in saying, *"Friend, give me three loaves"* (Luke 11:5).

Even in the Garden of Gethsemane, Jesus was specific: *"Take this cup from me."*

Why would this matter? Specific prayer is an opportunity for us to see God at work. Our faith grows when we see God responds in specific ways.

Specific prayer also lightens our burdens. Our anxieties threaten us because they are vague. When we are specific in our request to God, we reduce the problem to a prayer-size challenge.

"Cast your anxieties on God because He cares for you" (1 Peter 5:7), Scripture tells us.

Casting is an intentional act. Cast your troubles in God's hand; take your problems to God specifically and immediately. He promised to help you. Cling to his promises.

Why should we cast our anxieties to God? Because God cares *for us*! What a wonderful assurance! What a wonderful promise, isn't it? We need to cultivate the habit of being grateful instead of being fretful.

To pray is to remind God of His promise to help us. *"Put the Lord in remembrance* (of His promises), *keep not in silence"* (Isaiah 62.6), Scripture says.

"Put me in remembrance; let us contend together" (Isaiah 43:26), God told Isaiah.

"You said You would walk me through waters" (Isaiah 43:2), Isaiah reminded God. You said You would *"lead me through the valley"* {Psalm 23:4).

When you find yourself in the dark valley of life, remind God of His promise. *"You said You would never leave me or forsake me"* (Hebrews 13:5).

When you feel that God is far away or has abandoned you, remind Him of His promise not to forsake you.

Find a promise that fits your problem, then build your prayer around it. This kind of prayer of faith touches God's heart. Miracles will happen.

Remember, God will answer your prayer. God always answers our prayers. But God's answer may not coincide with what we expect. Trust God because He knows the future; we don't,

When I was a teenager, I had a crush on a girl who did not love me in return. I asked God to change the girl's heart to make her feel in love with me. At the time, I thought that she was the most precious thing in the world.

I prayed and fasted. But the girl did not have a change of heart.

In looking back, I thank God that she did not change her heart.

If she had fallen in love with me, I would have missed all the opportunities and blessings God had showered on me.

If you want peace in your life, if you want few anxious thoughts, fill your mind with Godly thoughts. Pray and the peace of God will guard your heart and mind.

CHAPTER 18

The secret of a contented life

Concerned about my well-being, some of my family members and friends told me that my wife would be better off in a nursing facility under the care of professionals because I am not trained or equipped to take care of her.

I am truly grateful for their concern. They are worried that I might lose my marbles or that in giving care, I might break my back, or become a victim of depression.

At first, I believed them but now, I don't.

Since having a stroke several years ago, she has been hospitalized four times and been in three different rehab facilities. The quality of care in these places was sub-standard compared to the care I am giving her, though I have no training for it.

After my horrible experiences at those facilities, I have concluded that as long as I am able, I will take care of my wife at home instead of putting her in a nursing home.

And she agrees. She is scared that something might happen that would make me unable to take care of her.

"I am sorry that your golden years are not golden," one of my daughters told me.

That may be true, but I would not be able to live with myself if it were any other way.

Thanks to God our Father for showering me with the graces I need to fulfill the difficult assignment He has given me and for providing me with a good teacher and a model in St. Paul, who guides me and teaches me the secret of how to find contentment in my golden years.

All of us seek contentment, but it is elusive.

Do you know what is the No.1 killer of contentment? I believe it is the "if only" lens of viewing life. "I would be content if only I was born taller or bigger" or "if only I was born rich" or "if only I had this or that talent."

"If only the kids would come" or "if only the kids were gone" or "if only my wife did not have a stroke."

Is "if only" a dominant factor in your life? If it is, you need to pay attention to St. Paul, who says *"A good life begins, not when circumstances change, but when our attitude to them does."*

Paul gives is an antidote to anxiety: *"Be anxious for nothing, but in everything, by prayer and supplication, with thanksgiving, let your request be known to God; and the peace of God, which surpasses all understanding, will guide your hearts and minds through Christ Jesus"* (Philippians 4:6-7).

Embedded in Paul's admonition are two beautiful words: **"*Thank you.*"**

Gratitude is one of the greatest virtues one can acquire. Gratitude is simply a mindful awareness of the benefits of life.

Studies show that gratitude has positive effects in one's life and that grateful individuals tend to be empathetic and more forgiving of others, have a more positive outlook on life and demonstrate less envy, materialism and self-centeredness.

Studies also show that gratitude improves self-esteem and enhances good relationships, quality of sleep and longevity. If gratitude were a pill, it would be considered a miracle cure.

An anxious heart says "I would be OK if I had this or that." A grateful heart says "Father God, You already have given me already this or that. Thank you, Father."

Stop and think of the blessings God has showered on you: family, friends, gifts, talent, skills and opportunities.

When you count your blessings, anxieties leave your heart. Anxiety and gratitude do not like each other.

You will be more content if you focus more on what you have and less on what you don't.

Imitate St. Paul, who said *"I have learned to be content whatever the circumstances. I know what it is to be in need and I know what it is to have plenty. I have learned the secret in being content in any and every situation, whether well-fed or hungry, whether living in plenty or in want. I can do all this through him who gives me strength* (Philippians 4:11– 13).

Paul wrote this exhortation while he was in jail. He was in a miserable situation. under constant surveillance and without hope for release. He was shackled. And yet he was able to say

"*I have learned the secret of being content.*" Paul was content in spite of his dire condition.

Did you notice this? Paul did not say "I have learned the principle" or "I have learned the concept." Instead, he said "*I have learned the secret.*"

A secret is a bit of knowledge not commonly known. Paul learned the secret of being content whether he was well-fed or hungry, in abundance or in need.

The secret of your contentment does not depend on the car you drive, the clothes you wear or how much you have in the bank. You cannot win in the rat race of materialism. There will always be nicer cars to drive and nicer clothes to wear.

Since the rat race is unwinnable, it creates a lot of anxieties. If you define yourself by how much stuff you have, you will feel good if you have a lot and you will feel bad if you don't have much.

Paul learned to be content with what he had. He was content with a jail instead of a house; he had four walls instead of a mission field; chains instead of jewelry; a guard instead of a wife.

Paul was content because he focused on eternal life, on the love of God, on forgiveness of sins.

Paul had Christ and that was enough. What he had in Christ was better than what he did not have in life: "*To me, the most important thing about living is Christ and dying would be profit for me*" (Philippians 1:21).

Paul's secret of contentment was to view life through a different lens – the lens of eternity.

Paul's only aim was to know Jesus. He was not attracted to riches. Applauses did not matter to him. Death did not scare him. All he wanted was more of Christ.

In Christ, we have contentment. Since no one can take Christ from us, no one can take our contentment.

If we are with Christ, death, sin, betrayal, sickness and disappointment cannot take our contentment from us.

Death cannot take our contentment. Christ is greater than death.

Sin cannot take our contentment. Christ is greater than sin.

Betrayal cannot take our contentment. Christ will never betray us.

Sickness cannot take our contentment. God has promised to heal us on either this side of the grave or the other side.

Disappointment cannot take our contentment. Although our plans may not work, God's plan will.

Christ is greater than anything you don't have in life. You have a God Who is crazy about you, a God Who watches and portects you. You have a God Who lives in your heart. In Christ, you have everything.

Anchor your life in the character of God. Moods will come and go. Situations will fluctuate. In Christ, your contentment will endure the storm of life.

If you want to be content, leave the "if only" lens of viewing life behind you. Look at what you already have; replace your anxious thoughts with greatful ones; deal with the cards in your hand. Bloom wherever you are planted.

CHAPTER 19

Do you know God in your heart?

"Oh my Lord, please stop her from calling me so many times. I need to sleep," I prayed.

"I have been pushing the red button several times, but nobody is coming to help me," my wife distressfully explained.

There was nothing I could do. The doors at her rehab facility are closed at 10 p.m.

I wanted to tell her that the world would not end if it took a while for the nurse to come help her. But I refrained.

That was only the beginning of a stormy day. In the morning when I started to leave home to go to the rehab center, my car did not start. The battery was dead. I proceeded to the other car. It had a flat tire.

Have you had this kind of day, when you just want to cry, put your hands up and say "I cannot take it anymore!"

But as I thought about it, the storm that hit me on that day was not as ferocious as those others have gone through.

I thought of John, who buried his wife the other day; of Rita, whose doctor told her that the cancer on her breast has metastasized; of Jennifer, whose husband left her for another woman, leaving her with three little boys to raise by herself.

We ask ourselves, "How on earth can we survive the storms in the ocean of life?"

St. Paul has a concise and profound answer to the question: *"The peace of God, which surpasses all understanding, will guard your hearts and minds through Christ Jesus"* (Philippians 4:7).

The peace of God is what we need when a storm hits us. Storms are unavoidable in our journey through the ocean of life. It is not a matter of "if," but "when."

What is this "peace of God" that Paul is talking about? It is not a peace *from* God; rather, it is God's peace; it is not a tranquility from God; rather, it is God's tranquility.

One night when the Apostles and Jesus were traveling across the Sea of Galilee, a ferocious storm hit their boat. The Apostles were so scared that they woke Jesus up, saying, "Jesus, we are perishing!"

"Why are you afraid? You know I am here!" Jesus told them.

He commanded the storm to quit and it did.

"Be still and know that I am God," the Psalmist says. Do you know God? I am sure you know Him in your head. But do know Him in your heart?

Not long ago, I saw a little boy and his father playing in a park. The boy was on a high platform, telling his dad, "Go farther," then jumping into his father's arms. The boy was not afraid to jump because he knew his father had strong arms.

What is "God's peace" like? It looks like this: We should be worried, but we are not; we should be upset, but we are not: we should be disappointed, but we are not.

God's peace transcends logic. We cannot explain it. God's peace is what sustained martyrs during their trials.

St. Lawrence was burned to death. "Turn me over. This side is already well done," he joked to his executioners.

St. Thomas More became weak while in prison and asked his executioners to help him climb up to the scaffold. He moved his beard away from the blade so it would not be cut. "Do not cut my beard. It did not commit treason," he humorously said.

St. Felicity fixed her hair before she entered the arena to be eaten by wild beasts. "I do not want people to think that I was grieving while waiting to die," she told her executioners.

During the Spanish civil war, hundreds of nuns were martyred and sang hymns on their way to their deaths.

God's peace is not a human achievement, but a peace from above. *"Peace I will live with you; my peace I give you. I do not give to you as the world gives. Do not let your hearts be troubled and do not be afraid"* (John 14:27), Scripture says.

It is the peace that calmed Jesus' heart when he was falsely accused; it is the peace that steadied his voice when he spoke to Pilate; it is the peace that kept his thoughts calm and his heart pure as he hung on the cross.

This peace can be ours, too. It guards our mind and our heart, through Christ Jesus (Philippians 4:7).

When we give ourselves to God, God takes responsibility for our hearts, our minds and our lives. God will do everything to bring us home to our Father's house. He will take all the steps to bring us home except one. He will allow us the freedom to make a choice.

Think about it. We do not have many choices in the important things in life. We did not choose our parents and siblings are; we did not choose the color of our skin; we did not choose the color of eyes or the size of our nose.

But we have a choice of where we spend eternity. Isn't that amazing?

You are the Lord's sheep: *"I am the good shepherd; I know sheep and my sheep know me* (John 10:14).

You are God's child and God is your Father: *"You are no longer a slave, but God's own child and since you are God's child, God made you His heir"* (Galatians 4:7).

You can have peace in the storm because you are not alone. You belong to God. Because we belong to God, we can have peace in the storm.

The same Jesus who sent an angel to Paul sends this message to you: *"When you pass through the waters, I will be with you"* (Isaiah 43:2).

When you face a perfect storm, Jesus will offer you a perfect peace.

CHAPTER 20

Thoughts Matter

"I hate going out!" my wife tells me every time she needs to leave the house for a doctor's appointment or to have her hair or nails fixed or for other activities that require leaving the house.

She hates to go out because she can no longer dress herself or go to her closet on her own to pick what she wants to wear.

Her inability to do the things she used to do before she became bedridden drives her nuts. I can understand her frustration. Can you? I could not imagine how I would feel if I could not dress myself.

Sometimes she vents her frustration on me and calls me names. This reopens deep wounds I endured as a little boy when I was bullied by older kids in our neighborhood.

"Shrimp!" I was called by the older boys, who made me cry and seemed to enjoy it. I tried to avoid them as much as possible, but it seemed they always caught up with me.

I became very timid. I believed that I was not as good as the kids who were older and bigger than me. I developed an inferiority complex.

One afternoon, Mrs. Apalisok, my Grade 4 teacher, saw me crying at the beginning of the class. When class was over, she took me to her office and asked why I was crying.

I shared my pain with her. "No way! You are not a shrimp; you are a mighty mite," she said, looking me in the eye and speaking with great seriousness, emphasis and authority.

"What is a mighty mite?" I asked.

"Something very small but powerful," she told me.

I started to believe what she said and it was amazing! When I started thinking of myself as a "mighty mite," I began to develop a sense of confidence. I started standing up to the bigger boys and in a few weeks, many of them became my friends and allies.

I wonder what would have happened if I did not have that conversation with Mrs. Apalisok. Looking back, it changed the trajectory of my life.

Was it grace? Or was it a miracle? Whatever it was, praise the Lord!

Mrs. Apalisok taught me that thoughts matter; that positive thoughts are good and that negative thoughts are bad.

This is an important concept. As Scripture warns us: "Be careful of what you think, because your thoughts run your life" (Proverbs 4:23).

"Most of our anxious feelings are caused by our irrational thoughts," said Dr. Albert Ellis, the founder of rational therapy.

The goal of rational therapy is to get rid of the irrational thoughts that produce anxiety.

St. Paul is a good rational therapist. He tells us, "Fix your thoughts on what is true and honorable, and the right and pure and lovely and admirable. Think about things that are excellent and worthy of praise" (Philippians 4:8).

Paul's point is simple: Face your anxiety with clear and logical thinking.

Thoughts matter, so be careful of what you are thinking. Be careful what kind of thoughts you allow to enter your mind. You have no choice in many things; you did not decide who your parents and siblings are; you did not determine your height or the size of your nose; you did not determine the amount of salt in the ocean; you cannot determine the weather. But you have a choice of what thoughts enter your head.

You are like an air traffic controller. You can control which thoughts land in and depart from your mind. No thought can enter your head without your permission.

If you want to be happy, you need to sow happy thoughts. It is in your power to control your thought pattern.

Do you want to be miserable? Then continue to wallow in the mud of self-pity, of guilt and of regrets. If you want to be miserable, assume the worst, beat yourself up and complain to those who listen to your whining.

The bigger problem is not your problem itself; rather, it is how you deal with your problem. Your greatest challenge is the manner in which you face your challenges.

The devil knows that thoughts matter, so he tries to mix your mind up by bombarding it with thoughts that carry fear and anxiety.

The devil tries to convince you to let bad thoughts enter your mind so they unload their stinking cargo and pollute your mind.

The devil comes like a thief with the sole intention of "stealing, killing and destroying" (John 10:10). He brings doom and gloom in our lives.

Do you remember Job? He was sick and felt abandoned after the devil was finished with him. Do you remember Judas? He hung himself after he had done what the devil told him to do.

Termites chew the wood from the inside. Similarly, the devil works from the inside of our mind.

The devil leads us to dark places and leaves us there to rot. The devil convinces us that the world has no windows; that there is no possibility of light to enter.

The devil specializes in exaggerations such as "No one will ever love you" or "It is all over for you" or "Everyone hates you" or "You will never have friends" or "You will never get out of debt."

The devil is a big liar. No problem is unsolvable; no life is irredeemable; no one is unlovable, even though the devil may convince you that you are unlovable.

Though the devil is a master of deceit, he is not a master of your mind. You have the power he cannot defeat. You have God on your side.

So fix your mind on what is true, honorable, right, pure, lovely and admirable.

"Capture every thought and make it give up and obey Christ" (2 Corinthians 10:5), Paul tells us. Guard your thoughts and learn to trust God.

Let us pray: "Father God, protect our mind from all schemes of the devil. We are thankful for our authority in Jesus; the devil has no lasting power over our mind! Please break any strongholds in the name of Jesus, bringing healing to my thought life. Please replace the devil's condemning voice with Your own and help us to be able to recognize his lies for what they are. Help us to grow in our knowledge of Your Word, so we can speak Your truth against his falsehoods. In Jesus' name, we pray. Amen."

CHAPTER 21

Don't let God's hand go

When my wife fell and fractured a bone on her left arm, she was hospitalized for three weeks and spent another three weeks at a rehab facility for physical and occupational therapy before she returned home.

I was always in both places because my wife had a difficult time doing things for herself with one arm. She needed help. Both places were understaffed; in both places, help was minimal.

While I was at these facilities, I observed that caregivers report to work at 7 in the morning, go home at 3 in the afternoon and are off during the weekend.

I was envious of their schedule. They work hard, but they have breaks.

I felt sorry for myself. I am on duty 24/7 with no weekends off.

"Poor me! I have a rotten life!" I told myself.

Negative thoughts flooded my mind: "I am like a prisoner. I have no time to do things for myself. I cannot leave the house for more than two hours."

How could I survive in my situation? Maybe I would have a nervous breakdown or a heart attack or a stroke.

I notice that caregiving is changing me. I am becoming a grumpy, cranky old man.

Thanks to God, I did not wallow long in the mud of self-pity. I thought of Mother Teresa of Calcutta. She worked tirelessly day in and day out, caring for the dying in the streets of Calcutta.

"How did Mother Teresa do it?" I asked myself.

While thinking of her work among the poor in Calcutta, I thought of the passage in Scripture where Jesus invites us to abide in Him.

"Abide in Me and I in you," Jesus invites us. "As the branch cannot bear fruit of itself, unless it abides in the vine, so neither can you, unless you abide in Me. I am the vine, you are the branches; he who abides in Me and I in him bears fruit, for apart from Me you can do nothing. If anyone does not abide in Me, he is thrown away as a branch and dries up; and they gather them and cast them into the fire, and they are burned. If you abide in Me and My words abide in you, ask and whatever you wish, it will be done for you. My Father is glorified by this, that you bear much fruit and so proved to be my disciples. Just as the Father has loved Me, I also have loved you. Abide in my love; just I have kept my Father's commandments and abide in His love" (John 15: 4 -10).

The allegory is simple: God is the vine keeper. Jesus is the vine and we are the branches.

The vine is the root and trunk of the plant. The root cables nutrients from the soil to the branches.

"I am the real root of life," Jesus claims. If anything good comes to our life, Jesus is the conduit.

"When we abide in Christ, we bear fruit: love, joy, peace, patience, kindness, goodness, faithfulness" (Galatians 5:22).

Jesus uses the word "abide" ten times in seven verses to make sure we do not miss His point.

"Come live with Me" or "Make my home your home," Jesus invites us.

Jesus does not say "I will check with you from time to time" or "I will visit you from time to time."

You know what it means to be at home. A home is not like a dorm room or a hotel room. Though a dorm room or a hotel room has beds and tables and other things we find at home, it is not a home.

To be at home is to feel safe. A home is a place of refuge. A home is a place of security. To be at home is to be comfortable.

Our primary goal in life is to be at home in Christ. Christ is our permanent residence. Christ is our mailing address.

We are familiar with the things at home. We do not need a blueprint to go the kitchen or bedroom. To be at home in Christ is to be familiar with Christ's attitude, heart and mind.

In Christ, we find rest. We find our nourishment in Him. His grace protects us from the storms of guilt. His providence shields us from life's destructive storms. His love warms us during life's lonely winters.

The branch's primary goal is to hang on to the vine. A healthy branch never releases the vine. Detached from the vine, the branch is dead.

Fruitfulness is not our main assignment. Faithfulness is. The secret to fruit bearing and anxiety-free living is less about doing and more about abiding.

"Abide in me" or "live with me" or "make my home your home," Jesus tells us.

Christians often talk about "changing the world" or "making a difference for Christ" or "leading people to the Lord." These are not goals. Rather, these are products of a Christ-focused life. These are fruits of abiding in Christ. A Christian's goal is to abide in Christ.

A Christian life is like a boy holding hands with his father as they cross a busy city street.

The father does not say "memorize the map" or "dodge the traffic" or "let us see if you could find your way home."

Rather, he says "hold on to me" or "hold my hand." The father gives the little boy one responsibility: "Hold my hand."

God our Father tells us to hang tightly to His hand as we cross the busy streets of life.

God is our good Father. God does not load us with a long list of responsibilities, with severe punishment for non-compliance. God does not demand that we know every detail of the future.

God gives us one goal: "Hold my hand and never let it go".

"Do not worry about your life or what you eat or drink; nor about your body, what you will put on" (Matthew 6:25), Jesus tells us.

And then Jesus gives us two commands: "look" and "consider."

Jesus commands us to look at the birds of the air.

When we look at the birds, we see that they seem happy. Have you seen a bird that is frowning, grumpy or cranky? "Watch the birds," Christ tells us. "The birds sing, whistle and soar. Yet the birds neither sow nor gather into barns."

"Consider the lilies in the field," Jesus commands us. The lilies don't do anything. God dresses them up for red-carpet appearances. Even the great king Solomon was not clothed like the lilies.

If God takes care of the birds and the lilies, will He not take care of us, too?

"If you abide in my word, you are truly my disciple and you will know the truth and the truth will set you free" (John 8: 31–32), Jesus says.

Free from what? Free from fear. Free from dread. And, yes, free from anxiety.

CHAPTER 22

You don't have to suck on your lemons

It started beautifully with hugs and kisses as we exchanged gifts. "My efforts paid off!" I said to myself. I was proud of myself for singly preparing a Christmas family party from scratch and in a limited time span.

The party was scheduled to start at 6 p.m. I left home for the grocery store at 10:30 a.m. to buy the things I needed to cook for the party, went to three different stores and had a difficult time finding the things I needed.

I then hurried home to start cooking. When I arrived, my wife needed personal assistance for her late-morning routine. I had no option but to help her with her basic needs. It was a huge interruption, but thanks to God, I was successful in maintaining my equilibrium.

I was like a duck which looks calm on the outside while its feet underneath in the water are furiously paddling.

With a knotted stomach, I had to fight the clock to accomplish my mission but I succeeded, though just barely.

Sadly, the party went sour and ended up with wounded hearts because politics was injected into it.

Former President Donald Trump was the bone of contention.

One faction was passionately for Trump and the other passionately against him.

Mea culpa! I should have stopped the argument before it hit the point of no return.

But the incident happened so fast that I did not have the opportunity to intervene. *Mea maxima culpa!*

Looking back, I wish I had not hosted the party, but then, "Why should I feel bad and anxious about what happened? How it ended was never a part of the plan," I rationalized.

I felt bad about the party but as with all my mistakes in the past, I could not undo it. All I could do was give it to the Lord.

"I will lift my eyes up to the hills; from whence comes my help? My help comes from the Lord, Who made heaven and earth" (Psalm 121:1-2.

Do not meditate about your mess. Do not set your eyes on your problem because you do not gain anything from doing so. Instead, lift up your eyes to the Lord.

This is a lesson Peter learned on the stormy Sea of Galilee. Peter was a fisherman. He knew what 10-foot waves could do to small boats.

Maybe that was why he jumped out of a little boat to reached out to Jesus, Who was walking on the waves during a fierce storm.

"Lord, is it really you?" Peter asked. "Then command me to come to you on the water."

"Come!" Jesus said.

Without thinking and without hesitation, Peter jumped from the boat and walked on water to Jesus.

But when Peter heard the wind and saw the waves, he became afraid and began to sink.

"Lord, save me!" Peter shouted (Matthew 14: 28–30).

Peter did the impossible as long as his eyes were focused on Christ's face. But when Peter removed his focus on Christ and looked at the storm instead, he sank like a piece of lead.

If you are sinking, like Peter, most probably your eyes are focused in the wrong direction.

If you feel that your problems are crushing you, maybe it is because you do not know or believe that God has complete control of the universe.

"God is the blessed controller of things, the King over all kings and Master of all masters," Scripture says (1 Timothy 6:15).

If God sustains and controls the whole universe, do you think that God cannot handle your problems? Do you think that God has no authority over your problems?

Are you depressed because of your sins? If you are, think about His mercy.

"There is now no condemnation for those who are in Christ Jesus," Scripture says (Romans 8:1).

Face God before you face your problems. Then ask God for help.

"Let your requests be known to God," Scripture says (Philippians 4:5).

Fear triggers either despair or prayer. Choose wisely.

"Come to Me in the time of trouble," God said (Psalm 50:15).

"Ask and it will be given to you; seek and you will find; knock and it will be opened to you," Jesus says (Matthew 7:7).

These promises of God do not have uncertainty. Jesus does not say "might" or "perhaps."

Jesus is unflinching. When you ask, He listens.

Jesus' message is simple: Leave your concerns with God. Let God take charge. Let God do what He is willing to do.

"Guard your hearts and minds through Jesus Christ" (Philippians 4:7).

When you go to a mechanic to have your car fixed, you drop it off and pick it up. You do not hang around and watch the mechanic do his job.

Our relationship with God is equally simple: Leave your problems with Him. "I know when I have believed and am persuaded that He is able to keep what I have committed to Him until that day" (2 Timothy 1:1-2). Paul reminds us.

God does not need either your advice or your help. Stop being God. God will tell you when He wants you to be involved with your problem again.

In the meantime, replace your anxious thoughts with grateful ones. God loves it when we are grateful to Him because when we are being grateful, we focus on the present.

Anxiety ruins our attention. Anxiety divides our mind; anxiety makes our awareness fly in many directions.

Anxiety makes us leave the present and look at the past, to the things we have done or said. It also makes us look to the future: What if I get sick or my car breaks down or I cannot find a job?

Leave your problems to God and meditate on good things.

"Finally, brethren, whatever things are true, whatever things are noble, whatever things are just, whatever things are pure, whatever things are lovely, whatever things are of good report, if there is any virtue and if there is anything praiseworthy – meditate on these things." Paul tells us (Philippians 4:8).

Do not let anxious and negative thoughts flood your mind. You cannot control the circumstances and situations, but you can control how you face them, you can control what you think of them.

"Lany, when you get a lemon, make a lemonade," my brother-in-law Jerry Crumpler used to tell me when I shared my problems with him.

Jerry knows that in the last few years of being a caregiver to his sister, I have been drinking plenty of lemonade. I know that the lemon supply is not scarce.

All of us drink lemonade because life gives lemons. Life gives lemons to good people and bad people, to young people and old people, to rich people and to poor people.

Thanks be to God, He does not require us to suck on them.

CHAPTER 23

Salute the process of life

It was a strange call. I did not expect it. It came from a funeral home, of all places. The individual on the other end of the line was trying to sell me a funeral package which could pay for my last expenses - my coffin and burial services.

The salesman was direct and to the point. After a very short pleasantry, he dropped the bomb on me.

"You know that funeral expenses are going up fast. Our company has a program with which you could pay for your funeral now at the current price," the salesman said. I thought it was a good idea, so I bought a package for my wife and myself.

He was not kidding and he was not laughing. It did not take a long time for him to convince me of the need for what he was selling.

I do not want to burden my children about my departure from this world.

'Before we finalize the deal, I would like to ask you a sensitive question. What do you want to wear when you are buried?" the salesman asked me.

"Barong Tagalog!" I responded.

Barong Tagalog is attire used in the Philippines in special occasions such as a wedding or a funeral. It is equivalent to a tuxedo in the United States.

Barong Tagalog is made of fine pineapple fiber.

The topic of death was never a part of the plan for this book. It was as it the funeral salesman made me do it.

Do not get an idea that I have a premonition of my own death or my wife's. I know that I am going die, but when I die is not my call. It's God's. God has not told me the date and I am not really interested in knowing.

Death could be defined as a birth to a new life. I like this definition.

Dr. Wayne Dyer tells this story in his book, *Your Sacred Self*:

In a mother's womb were two babies. One asked the other, "Do you believe in life after delivery?"

"Of course, there has to be something after delivery," the other responded. "Maybe we are here to prepare ourselves for what we will become later."

"Nonsense!" said the first. "There is no life after delivery. What kind of life would that be?"

"I do not know. But there will be more light than here. Maybe we will walk with our legs and eat with our mouths.

Maybe we will have other senses that we cannot understand now," the second said.

The first said, "That is absurd. Walking is impossible.

And eating with our mouths? That's ridiculous. The umbilical cord supplies nutrition and everything we need. But the umbilical cord is so short. Life after delivery is logically to be excluded."

The second insisted, "Well, I think there is something and maybe it is different than it is here. Maybe we do not need this physical cord anymore."

The first replied, "Nonsense! And moreover, if there is life, then why is it that no one has ever come back from there? Delivery is the end of life and after delivery there is nothing but darkness, silence and oblivion. It takes us nowhere."

The second said, "Well, I do not know. But certainly, we will meet Mother and she will take care of us."

The first replied, "Mother? You actually believe in Mother? That's laughable. If Mother exists, where is she now?

The second said. "She is all around us. We are surrounded by her. We are of her. It is in her that we live. Without her this world could not exist".

The first said. "Well, I don't see her, so it is only logical that she does not exist."

The second replied, "Sometimes when you are in silence and you focus and you really listen, you can perceive her presence and you can hear her loving voice, calling down from above."

Another story relates death from the viewpoint of a boy building a sand castle:

On his knees, he scoops up to and packs the sand with a plastic shovel into an orange bucket. Then he upends the bucket on the surface and lifts it, and to the delight of the little architect, a tower is created.

All afternoon he will work, spooning out the moat and packing the walls. Popsicle sticks will be the bridges. And a sand castle will be built.

He is diligent and determined. He knows that the tide will rise and the end of his castle will come as the sun sets. He knows that each wave slaps closer to his creation.

But the boy does not panic. He is not surprised. The pounding of the waves reminds him that the end of his creation is inevitable. He knows the secret of the surging.

As the waves near, the little boy jumps to his feet and begins to clap. He has no fear, no sorrow and no regrets. He knows the castle will be destroyed. He is not surprised.

When a great wave crashes into his masterpiece, it is sucked into the sea and he smiles, picks up his tools, takes his father's hand and goes home.

We can learn from the little boy about our own sand castles. Whatever we accomplish on this earth will end. Someday, like the boy, we will have to pick up our tools, hold our Father's hand and go home.

Like the little boy, we live with rhythmic reminders. Days come and go. Seasons ebb and flow. Every sunrise that turns to sunset whispers to us a secret: "Time will take our castle away."

Nobody knows when the day and the time will be – not even the angels of heaven, not even the Son. Only the Father knows (Matthew 24:36).

Jesus' message is unmistakable. He will return, but we know not when.

This is what Jesus tells us in the parable of the virgins (Matthew 25:1-13), the parable of the talents (Matt. 25:14-30) and the parable of the sheep and the goats (Matthew 25:36).

At times, we treat this world as our permanent home. Jesus reminds us that it is not.

Sometimes we pour energy and time into life on earth as though it will last forever. Jesus reminds us that it won't.

At times, we are proud of what we have done and hope never to leave it. Jesus reminds us that we will have to let it go. Jesus reminds us that we are transitory in this world.

I do not know much about sand castles, but children do. Jesus tells us to watch them and learn from them.

Jesus tells us to build our sand castles in life, but to build them with a child's heart and to applaud them when the sun sets and the tide takes them away.

Jesus tells us to salute the process of life, to take our Father's hand and go home.

CHAPTER 24

Thank you!

Dear Reader,

By reading *"Footprints in the Sand of Caregiving,"* I consider it as allowing me to share with you my struggles as a caregiver. I thank you for it. May God bless you for it.

Writing *"Footprints in the Sand of Caregiving"* was like therapy for me. It was a means for me to release the pressure of caregiving that was building in my heart.

Facing singly the challenges of 24/7 caregiving made my heart like a time bomb ready to explode. Writing my challenges down was like a release valve which slowed down the pressure-building process.

I post spiritual things on Facebook and write reflections on any platform available to me. Please understand that I am not trying to appear "holier than thou." Like everybody else, I fight temptations daily and fall from time to time.

Like everyone else, I am a piece of "work in progress." I am still confessing the same sins, though I vow to amend my life.

I am working on being more kind and more charitable. I still lose my temper. From time to time I still regress, I say unkind words or slam doors. Oh, yes, I still pout and my pouting drives my wife nuts.

My caregiving journey is still in progress. I do not know what the future will bring. I continue holding on to my Lord's hand for the days ahead.

I thank the Lord for His steadfast love; I thank Him for His mercies that are new every morning; I thank Him for His faithfulness.

Dear reader, again I thank you for reading the book. I commit my wife and me to your prayers, and be assured of our own for you.

May God bless you and your loved ones.

Hasta la vista, amigos and amigas.

Sincerely in Mary of Mount Carmel,
Lany

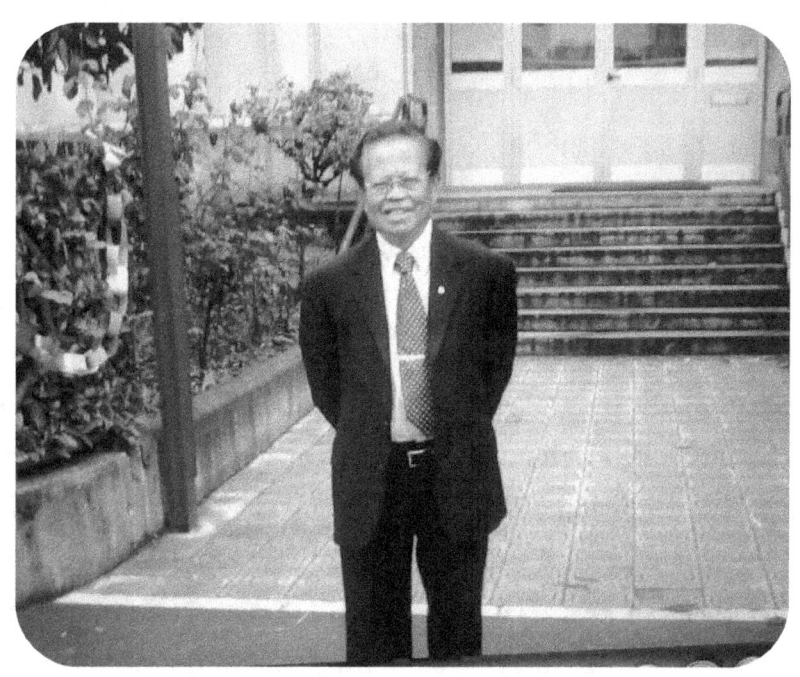

BIOGRAPHY

Leandro (Lany) Maniwang Tapay, a native of Balilihan, Bohol, Philippines. His pursuit of knowledge le earned a Bachelor's Degree in Education with a major in English and Spanish, along with a minor in Social Sciences. Embarking on further academic endeavors, he underwent Philosophical studies at Seminario de San Carlos in Cebu City and Don Bosco Seminary in Canlubang, Calamba, both in the Philippines. Continuing his theological studies abroad, he attended the Pontifical College Josephinum in Worthington, Ohio, USA. Notably, he expanded his expertise by earning a Master's Degree in Guidance and Counseling at the Ohio State University in Columbus, Ohio, USA. Leandro Maniwang Tapay's educational journey reflects a diverse and extensive commitment to learning across various disciplines and geographical locations.

Lany's professional journey extends beyond traditional teaching roles, encompassing a diverse range of responsibilities. He began by imparting knowledge of Religious courses at Cebu Boys' Town in Cebu City, Philippines, fostering spiritual growth among students. Transitioning to the United States, he undertook the position of teaching Latin and Religion Courses at Saint Mary High School in North Dakota, where he also served as the Dean of Boys at Saint Mary's boarding school.

His commitment to holistic education extended to Central Catholic School in Toledo, Ohio, USA, where he taught Christian Meditation courses, emphasizing the importance of contemplative practices. His dedication to education and guidance reached new heights as the Guidance Director at London High School in London, Ohio, demonstrating his proficiency in counseling and support for students.

In a testament to his dedication to education accessibility, Lany engaged in moonlighting as he taught Philosophy Courses at Urbana University's outreach program at the London Prison Facility, showcasing a commitment to extending education to diverse settings.

Additionally, Leandro took on the significant role of Diocesan Director of the Pontifical Mission Societies in the United States, Diocese of Columbus, demonstrating leadership in fostering mission-driven initiatives within the diocese.

Beyond his professional endeavors, Lany displayed a compassionate side as a 24/7 caregiver, showcasing his selfless commitment to the well-being of others. Through this multifaceted journey, Leandro has left an indelible mark not only as an educator but also as a caregiver and community leader.

www.ingramcontent.com/pod-product-compliance
Lightning Source LLC
LaVergne TN
LVHW010223070526
838199LV00062B/4703